Professional Issues in Child and Youth Care Practice

This book provides an overview of the core professional issues in the field of child and youth care practice. The author explores themes ranging from relationships and the exploration of Self to career building and field-specific approaches to management. The book is written from a pragmatic perspective, and serves both to advance current thinking in the field about professional issues as well as to provide the student of child and youth care practice and practitioners with practical and accessible approaches to developing a strong and sustainable professional identity. All of the themes in this book are explored within a context of ethical decision-making and practice approaches informed by a commitment to children's rights and empowerment. Throughout the discussions, concepts and themes are considered in relation to four specific lenses: the power lens, the diversity lens, the language lens and the transitioning from theory to practice lens. These lenses serve to ensure that the reader adopts a critical understanding of the professional issues in the field and is able to develop his or her own professional identity while mitigating the power and identity issues necessarily associated with being a practitioner in a helping profession.

This book was published as a special issue of *Child and Youth Services*.

Kiaras Gharabaghi is Assistant Professor in the School of Child and Youth Care at Ryerson University in Toronto, Canada, and has been involved in child and youth care practice for over twenty years.

Professional Issues in Child and Youth Care Practice

Kiaras Gharabaghi

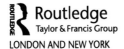 Routledge
Taylor & Francis Group

LONDON AND NEW YORK

First published 2010 by Routledge
2 Park Square, Milton Park, Abingdon, Oxon, OX14 4RN

Simultaneously published in the USA and Canada
by Routledge
270 Madison Avenue, New York, NY 10016

Routledge is an imprint of the Taylor & Francis Group, an informa business

This book is a reproduction of *Child & Youth Services*, vol. 30, issue 3-4. The Publisher requests to those authors who may be citing this book to state, also, the bibliographical details of the special issue on which the book was based

Typeset in Times by Value Chain, India
Printed and bound in Great Britain by
TJI Digital, Padstow, Cornwall

British Library Cataloguing in Publication Data
A catalogue record for this book is available from the British Library

ISBN10: 0-415-58297-0
ISBN13: 978-0-415-58297-1

Contents

ABSTRACTS

1. Professional Issues in Child and Youth Care

Several contexts and themes of professionalism are considered including the nature of "professional issues," professionalism, and writing about professional issues. The professional issues discussed are the socio-political and cultural contexts, systems, employment, career development, relationships with other professionals, and the self. Next, I discuss the professional issues of professional organization, arguing that the professional status of child and youth care matters less than the meaning of the work to practitioners. I also argue that more work needs to be done before the field can be professionally organized. Finally, I suggest both scholarly research work and less formal, more accessible writing have a rightful place in the ongoing evolution of the field.

2. Boundaries and the Exploration of Self

Boundaries and the exploration of self are conceptualized within the agency-structure problem first articulated in social theory during the 1970s. Constructing boundaries as a professional issue within the discipline has to take account the agency embedded within boundaries. Multiple boundary dilemmas are discussed within the framework of the agency-structure problem, including those that result from policies and procedures, and it is further argued that boundaries and the exploration of self also impact at the team level. Finally, the role of power imbalances within the practice of boundary formation is explored in relational worker–client interactions.

3. Values and Ethics in Child and Youth Care Practice

The implications of the practitioner's personal values are explored in relation to the professional issues of child and youth care practice.

Values are inevitably a component of decision-making and therefore are integrally connected to ethics in the field. The prevalence of subjectivity over objectivity is emphasized in relation to in-the-moment decision-making for practitioners. This results in an elevated importance for the process of critical reflection with respect to personal values. The ethics of child and youth care practice are explored from both systemic and in-the-moment perspectives. The role of codes of ethics is explored as well as ethics in relation to self care and professional development, everyday preparation and practice and ethics in relation to team dynamics and functioning.

4. Relationships with Children and Families

This article explores the professional issues of relationships within child and youth care practice. The concept of "relationship-based practice" is examined from conceptual, linguistic and power-based perspectives. It is argued that the power base of relationships amongst practitioners manifests itself along five specific contexts: institutional dynamics, culture, conventions, social expectations, and language. Relationship-based practice is compared with relational practice. It is argued that a more complex view of relationships within child and youth care practice will serve to prevent misuses and poorly defined practices on the part of practitioners. To this end, it is recommended that greater emphasis be placed within the discipline on the relational content of training and professional development activities.

5. Relationships Within and Outside of the Discipline of Child and Youth Care

This article explores the practitioner's relationships with colleagues, on teams and with professionals from other disciplines and systems. While there has been much analysis and discussion about relationships between practitioners and clients, there has been relatively little attention paid to the professional relationships that are at the center of the practitioner's day-to-day work. It is within these relationships that practitioners encounter both opportunities and challenges in positioning themselves effectively to deliver a positive service to clients. As such, in this article are descriptions of the relationships amongst child and youth care practitioners, between practitioners and other professionals as well as between practitioners and other systems. Several core themes are identified including the importance of communication and networking as well as the role of power imbalances in defining the nature of such relationships.

6. The Community Context of Child and Youth Care Practice

Child and youth care practice unfolds within the context of the community. It is therefore essential that practitioners develop reflective skills not only in relation to their clients and the organizational context in which they are employed, but also in relation to their presence within a community and the community's perception of the practitioner's presence. The role of community within child and youth care practice is explored in relation to the professional issues that can arise for practitioners. It is argued that practitioners both use and contribute to the communities in which they work and that, therefore, an active engagement with communities will require the practitioner to be aware of the implications of their presence with respect to culture, power and community conventions. Finally, the possibility of expanding the role of the practitioner to incorporate community capacity building is also explored. Child and youth care practice is ideally situated to contribute proactively to community capacity as in most communities, capacity issues are very much related to living with children and youth.

7. Professional Issues of Child and Youth Care Through the Language Lens

This article explores the role of language and forms of communication in professional child and youth care practice. It is argued that all the professional issues of child and youth care practice are significantly impacted by language and the manner in which practitioners use language and a variety of communication forms to articulate their work. The role of jargon in child and youth care practice is examined using several commonly used terms as examples. The need for an ongoing, critical perspective in the use of language is emphasized, and practitioners are encouraged to contemplate the biases and unexamined truths embedded in their day-to-day language use.

8. Professional Development and Career Building in Child and
Youth Care

This article explores the current status of professional development within
the child and youth care field. Pre-service, inservice and professional
development activities and systems are critically examined in residential
and nonresidential contexts, and barriers to more effective training within
the field are identified. While there has been considerable effort both in
terms of research and practice with respect to pre-service curriculum
development, it is argued that in-service training for practitioners is sparse,
often random and rarely coordinated to meet the knowledge and skill needs
of practitioners relative to their specific employment context. Foundational
elements for career building in child and youth care are also explored,
and it is argued that notwithstanding virtually unlimited opportunities for
career building and the expansion of the field, there are some areas of
practice that are beyond the scope of the child and youth care profession.
Particular emphasis is placed on some of the contradictions between child
and youth care theory and practice fields such as child protection, therapy
and diagnostic work.

9. Child and Youth Care Approaches to Management

This article explores the themes and issues related to child and youth
care approaches to management. The profession is significantly
underrepresented at the management level. To some extent, this
reflects the challenges of being recognized in the broader human
services sector as a profession, but perhaps more so, it reflects an
underdevelopment of skills, knowledge and managerial pragmatism
on the part of the practitioner. It is argued that management customs
and requirements place child and youth care values and principles at
risk. However, there are steps that can be taken to mitigate such risks.
Common themes and processes of management roles are discussed
including performance management, orientation, recruitment and
supervision. Child and youth care practitioners are ultimately
well placed to assume management positions in residential and
nonresidential contexts but, in so doing, they must ensure that their
managerial identity maintains the fundamental values and principles
of the discipline.

ACKNOWLEDGEMENTS

This book represents the many lessons I have learned during my twenty plus years of practice in the field of child and youth care. I would have learned nothing at all were it not for the courage of the children, youth and families I encountered along the way, as well as the many child and youth care practitioners who have inspired me.

I would like to thank Doug Magnuson for his support, gentle critique and editorial work on this book. I am also grateful to my students Kim Speed and Karen Eacott, who worked hard under tight deadlines to provide me with literature finds and student perspective. It may not have been the most pleasant time in their lives but I hope the effort was worth it.

Several friends and colleagues have shaped my thinking and motivated me to continue thinking over the past few years: a heartfelt thank you to Bill Carty, Thom Garfat and Carol Stuart.

Ultimately I am forever in debt to my own family for allowing me the indulgence of writing about my thoughts. I therefore dedicate this book to Patti, Alex, Jett and Siena.

Professional Issues in Child and Youth Care

SUMMARY. Several contexts and themes of professionalism are considered including the nature of "professional issues," professionalism, and writing about professional issues. The professional issues discussed are the socio-political and cultural contexts, systems, employment, career development, relationships with other professionals, and the self. Next, I discuss the professional issues of professional organization, arguing that the professional status of child and youth care matters less than the meaning of the work to practitioners. I also argue that more work needs to be done before the field can be professionally organized. Finally, I suggest both scholarly research work and less formal, more accessible writing have a rightful place in the ongoing evolution of the field.

KEYWORDS. Child and youth care professional issues, social and cultural contexts, career development, inter-professional relationships, child and youth care employment issues, professionalization, professional organization, youth development, professional development

It is a strange profession indeed when one of the great contributors of knowledge within the profession, Henry Maier, apparently felt it necessary to remind child and youth workers that one of the things they ought to do each day is "say hello" to the children and youth they work with (Maier, 2003). One would not think that it is necessary for child and youth care practitioners to be reminded of such a basic element of civilized human interaction. In fact, one would expect a professional in the field of child and youth care practice to say hello and a whole bunch more to clients as a matter of course. But such is the nature of what we do; it ranges from the seemingly obvious to the banal to the sophisticated and all the way to the apparently insane. Jack Phelan (2008) exclaimed during a conference presentation that "What child and youth care workers do is simple, but their rationale for doing so is complex."

Child and youth care is a label that captures a wide range of activities. Such activities include those that are action-oriented, concrete and relatively easily understood by those who might inquire about them as well as activities that are seemingly passive, that lack any discernible movement or action, and that are much more difficult to explain to others who might be interested. It is one thing to say that we work with children and youth and that our work might include therapeutic play and problem-solving and behavior modification. While each of these terms is rendered meaningful through the interpretations and perspectives of those exposed to them, at least there is an element of visualization that can unfold within a general context of such activities (VanderVen, 2003). On the other hand, when we say that child and youth work is about "being" with children and youth and about developing relationships with them, we quickly move from somewhat comprehensible ideas to language that seems to suggest that child and youth care is really about not much of anything. As Fewster (1982) put it more than 25 years ago, "It's not very impressive ... to build a professional identity around the simple ability to relate to kids. Understanding how a particular child sees himself or the world around him is not likely to impress the neighbors or command respect within the professional community."

What child and youth workers do and what they are thought to be doing by others are often two completely different things (Weisman, 1999). Furthermore, most child and youth workers are themselves unsure about what it is they do, but they are busy doing a lot. Paradoxically, it has become increasingly difficult to find common understandings of what child and youth care is precisely at a time when child and youth workers are working in more service sectors than ever before.

This series of articles explores this and other professional issues of child and youth care practice. The exploration is informed by the ever-increasing divide between the development of the discipline of child and youth care in academic and research contexts on the one hand, and the evolution of the profession in the field, in agencies, in communities and in the minds of the practitioners on the other hand (Gannon, 2003; Stuart, 2008; Winfield, 2005). While this divide is not often acknowledged, when it is, the message is clear. As Phelan (2000) put it: "I am worried that the writers and teachers whom I talk to only really make sense to other writers and teachers, not actual practitioners. New staff, and especially students in field placement, quickly abandon all theoretical concepts in the face of the sensory overload that immobilizes them as they start to work in residential group care. There often is a lot of support from less skilled staff to do this and to start using 'common sense' approaches."

I want to contemplate the possibilities for the future of the profession, the dilemmas faced by practitioners in the present and some of the core themes that are and will continue to impact on the development of the profession and on the development of the practitioners, including themes of power, language and diversity. Such an exploration and contemplation requires a degree of flexibility in how we articulate thoughts and ideas; I will present these in both theoretical and conceptual terms, but I will also present these in pragmatic and extremely practical terms. And rather than moving from theory to practice or vice versa, I will move between theory and practice without warning and without missing a beat.

In writing these articles, I am reminded of a scene in a really bad 1980s movie starring Rodney Dangerfield. Dangerfield plays a character who returns to college after having successfully built a business empire in the oversized clothing industry. In one scene, Dangerfield interrupts the highly trained and educated professor who is lecturing on business principles, and he begins to provide his version of business principles that include such things as bribing city officials in order to get some breaks on garbage disposal regulations, manipulating tax accountants, aggressively pursuing personal relationships with potential business partners, and so on. The professor is disgusted by this presentation, but all the other students are eagerly taking notes, ignoring the professor's lecture and focusing on the much more practical and "real world" knowledge being shared by Dangerfield.

I aim for somewhere between the professor's and Dangerfield's versions of how to conduct business. On the one hand, there is today a great deal of academic work—conceptual and research based—that can in fact advance the professional context in which child and youth care practitioners do their work. On the other hand, the everyday experience of child and youth care practitioners is not quite as clean, not quite as controlled, and not quite as simple as it is presented in much of our academic discussions. Therefore, my approach to writing these articles has been one that tries to speak to the everyday realities facing practitioners while, at the same time, I have tried to contribute to the academic discussions about specific topics and themes as well. My hope is that the reader will find something startling, upsetting, and thought-provoking for discussion with colleagues, friends, children and youth, as well as professors and teachers. Before I embark on this exploration of the professional issues of child and youth care, it is worthwhile to clarify what I mean by professional issue, as well as to review, ever so briefly, some of the discussions and debates about professional issues in our field that I will not cover in the articles to come.

WHAT IS A PROFESSIONAL ISSUE

When one uses the term "professional issue," it begs the question how such an issue is differentiated from other kinds of issues. After all, we do commonly use terms such as "clinical issues," "practice issues," "research issues" and "personal issues" as well. Conversely, why are we talking about professional *issues* as opposed to professional solutions, problems, themes or approaches? It is difficult to provide clear and concrete answers to any of these questions. It is probably fair to say that there are no clear separations between professional and clinical issues, or between professional issues and professional approaches, solutions or themes. The first conclusion we can therefore draw is that any discussion or contemplation about professional issues that we might engage in represents an approximation more so than a determination; we are contemplating something that we can define within rather broad parameters only, recognizing that the designation of something as a professional issue is not really a scientific or even particularly firm categorization but, instead, a loose and pragmatic designation that neither is nor has to be consistently maintained.

With these limitations in mind, we can nevertheless propose a working definition of "professional issues" that at least will guide us through this series of articles and that might explain why some topics are covered and others are not. For the purpose of these articles, therefore, a professional issue is one that meets some, most or all of the following criteria:

- Societal, cultural and political issues that impact or potentially impact on the practitioner;
- Issues that reflect the systems context in which child and youth care practitioners operate;
- Issues that reflect the employment context of child and youth care practitioners;
- Issues that reflect the career development prospects of child and youth care practitioners;
- Issues that reflect the interactions of practitioners with professionals within the field or from other fields;
- Issues that are fundamentally about the practitioner, even if they manifest themselves within the context of the practitioner "being" with a child, youth or family.

This list of criteria is far from exhaustive, but it does cover a wide range of issues, themes and scenarios that constitute a frame of reference for contemplating the profession of child and youth care practice and the professional identity of the child and youth care practitioner. It is worthwhile, therefore, to provide some examples for each of these criteria so that, as we move forward in our contemplation of the professional issues in child and youth care practice, we have some idea about the limitations of what we will cover and the opportunities for reflection on issues left unexplored.

Society, Culture and Politics

Historically, child and youth workers were somewhat insulated from the broader societal, cultural and political dynamics of their work (Ingram & Harris, 2001). The institutions that typically employed child and youth workers frequently were closed off to the public, including particular communities, neighborhoods and even families. As a result, the social, cultural and political experience of child and youth workers was reflective of the subcultures and politics prevalent within their work settings. Of course, these subcultures and politics were themselves influenced by broader societal dynamics, but there was little emphasis on understanding the relationship between what is "out there" to what happens "in here."

All of this has changed considerably over the past two or three decades. De-institutionalization has resulted in the deployment of child and youth workers in much more open settings, even in the context of residential care. Group homes and residential treatment centers, as well as shelters and drop in programs for homeless youth, are now commonly located in neighborhoods and communities with no specific access barriers beyond security related measures to prevent unwanted intruders. Child and youth workers now have to deal with neighborhood concerns, changes in the community and patterns of violence and crime in spaces where they work. As the profession has moved beyond its historical focus on residential care, child and youth workers doing family work in private homes or providing services in community centers and other public spaces now are impacted by the social, political and cultural context of their employment spaces, and this has raised myriad professional issues for the discipline that were less obvious and perhaps less prevalent in the past.

Increasing diversity and acknowledgement of that diversity has resulted in a focus on anti-oppression approaches to being with children and youth as well as issues of racism and other forms of discrimination that are more openly identified and debated not only in the context of the specific services being provided but also in the context of relationships between staff, organizational dynamics and employment standards (Moore, 2001; Ragg, Patrick, & Ziefert, 2006; Skott-Mhrye, 2006). Issues of poverty and social alienation amongst particular demographic groups, especially in urban areas, has resulted in greater attention to social phenomena such as youth gangs, gun violence, drug trafficking and other issues that raise both safety-related concerns for practitioners as well as questions about cultural competence and ethical commitments in terms of working with clients without becoming an inadvertent informant for the local crime stopper program (Finlay, 2007; Gharabaghi, 2005; Schissel, 1997).

The politics of justice have intruded significantly in the employment environments of many child and youth workers. A "get tough on crime" mentality frequently promoted by government and citizen groups alike has impacted on the integrity of the child and youth care approach, which tends to prioritize relationships and caring over investigating wrong doing and convicting the perpetrators. Canada, for example, has the highest rate of youth incarceration amongst the OECD countries, and this is reflected in the large number of criminal charges emerging out of environments where child and youth workers are employed, notably of course residential care facilities (Finlay, 2007).

Other issues, including employment equity, unionization, accountability and transparency, all have become much more prevalent in recent years and have impacted the professional experiences of practitioners (Ingram & Harris, 2001). It is therefore critically important that when one considers the professional issues of child and youth care practice, one is conscious of the broader social, political and cultural dynamics unfolding locally, nationally and even globally. It is simply no longer possible to fully appreciate the full complexity of professional issues based on an analysis of the day-to-day experience of child and youth workers in their sometimes insular work environments.

Systems Context

In most jurisdictions in North America and, perhaps to a lesser extent in Europe, the issues and needs of children and youth are serviced by a fragmented and frequently uncoordinated system of service providers, service sectors and funding streams. While much of the literature and theory of child and youth care, social pedagogy and other human services fields have long recognized the interconnectedness of issues and themes faced by children and youth as well as their families, the response to such issues is parceled out between entirely separated institutional service providers in sectors such as education, child welfare, youth justice and others.

As a result, children and youth encountered by practitioners frequently have been or still are involved in helping systems beyond that in which any particular practitioner is employed. This, in turn, places considerable onus on the child and youth workers to be knowledgeable of other systems and to maintain extraordinarily high standards with respect to professional communication across sectors and service providers, participation in multi-sectoral and multi-disciplinary case management processes as well as advocacy to assist clients in navigating the full complexity of an uncoordinated and often rather expansive system of services. It also creates challenges for the practitioner to follow through on some of the more fundamental conceptual components of the discipline such as, for example, being with children and youth in their life spaces. Given the bureaucratic nature of virtually all of the sectors and service providers involved with the children and youth, accessing these spaces for any particular practitioner is often not so easy. Jurisdictional conflict, agency territorialism, and professional arrogance on the part of individuals or agencies are formidable obstacles to providing a service to children and youth that transcends these systemically entrenched but highly artificial separations and divides. Client files are transferred between sectors and institutions based on events and scenarios in the present, resulting in a watering down of responsibility and accountability for outcomes on the part of any single service provider or practitioner. The classic example, of course, is that of youth criminal justice. A youth living in a group home is transferred to a custody facility after committing a crime, and rather than a continued and seamless relational response from the child and youth care practitioners in the group home, the lifespace reality of that youth is now shifted entirely to the new setting where another team of child and youth workers engages the youth anew.

The systems context of child and youth care practice is clearly not one designed by the profession. Instead, it is one driven in part by funding streams and bureaucratic considerations far removed from the everyday practice of child and youth care workers. As such, this systems context presents child and youth workers with myriad professional issues that are sometimes difficult to resolve entirely.

The Employment Context

Never has the employment context of child and youth care practice been as complex as it is today. This reflects, in part, the ever-increasing sectors and institutions interested in hiring child and youth care practitioners, but it also reflects changes in the expectations of newly emerging generations of practitioners. Whereas in the past, a commitment to group care was really the primary requirement for practitioners to become engaged in the profession, today practitioners have choices and opportunities that simply were not available before. The prospects of low pay, difficult schedules and often turbulent day-to-day work experiences are now juxtaposed with the possibilities of steady schedules, better pay and greater professional recognition in sectors such as education, health care and clinical intervention settings specializing in group work or treatment approaches to specific conditions or disorders.

All of this has placed pressure on service settings to engage with practitioners on issues of material compensation and working conditions, an engagement that is in many cases mediated by unions. It has also created a wide range of professional issues for practitioners in terms of pre-service qualifications, opportunities for professional development, career development incentives and competition.

At the same time, the employment context of child and youth care practitioners has evolved into much more formalized and bureaucratic institutions and organizations, with reporting responsibilities and externally conducted audits and inspections. This, in turn, has impacted on the nature of policies and procedures guiding the day-to-day work of child and youth workers, with new regulations and sometimes difficult to manage expectations in terms of boundaries, program design and behavior management strategies.

The funding context of employers has increasingly been destabilized as well, resulting in a greater number of child and youth care positions being hired "on contract" or in the form of casual or relief-based employment. This too impacts on the practitioner in many different ways. Certainly one outcome is that often a practitioner has less loyalty for his or her specific employment context and is always on the lookout for more permanent and secure positions elsewhere. It also has created a whole new breed of child and youth worker that is not employed on a full-time basis anywhere but that maintains multiple part-time or contract positions across sectors with many different employers. This type of child and youth worker creates a new set of professional issues that range from a lack of supervision to a lack of training to a lack of accountability sometimes with very negative outcomes for children and youth.

Career Development Prospects

There has been much discussion in the field of child and youth care that pertains to lateral movement with respect to career development. Less discussed has been the issue of vertical movement and, specifically, management-related career aspirations of practitioners. Traditionally, management positions have been considered primarily in a residential context where child and youth care practitioners have frequently been hired into supervisory positions. A rich literature on supervision already exists (Delano, 2001; Garfat, 2001; Magnuson & Burger, 2001; Maier, 1985; Mann-Feder, 2001; Phelan, 1990; Ricks, 1989) but very little has been written about managerial positions outside of the residential context. In fact, management-related topics are typically discussed within the broader subfield of child and youth care administration, with often implicit assumptions that such administration is carried out by other professionals, impacting child and youth care practitioners working front line. It is, however, increasingly necessary to consider the prospects of child and youth care practitioners as managers, involved not only in the supervision of other child and youth care practitioners but also in dynamics such as program design and development, human resource management and the supervision of professionals from other fields.

The core professional issues that arise for child and youth care practitioners hired into management positions is how to maintain the integrity of the discipline while carrying out functions that have not traditionally been based on the core concepts of the field. Specifically, the relational characteristic of the profession is easily displaced by the pragmatic and outcome-oriented approaches of human resource managers and other administrators. And yet, much like we were able to incorporate child and youth care principles and approaches into some of the newly available front-line positions, such as family work (Garfat, 2003), it is also possible to incorporate such principles and approaches into the context of management positions. For the practitioner, balancing career aspirations with maintaining professional integrity raises a host of professional issues that will have to be contemplated and examined.

Relationships with Other Professionals

Perhaps one of the more obvious places to look for professional issues in the discipline is in the context of child and youth worker relationships with other professionals, including other child and youth workers. It is in this context that the professional identity of the practitioner is at its most vulnerable. Interactions with other professionals expose our weakness: talking about what we do, articulating our strategies and approaches, and—following the phrasing of Jack Phelan mentioned earlier—framing our simple activities within the full complexity of their rationale. It is also within this context that the practitioner is exposed to some of the deeply-held anxieties and vulnerabilities that come with working in a field that has not yet been fully recognized as a really professional field and that has, in fact, not fully established even within itself its professional credentials.

An additional challenge faced by many practitioners in their relationships with other professionals is that child and youth care practice is almost never a mandated service, in contrast to what police officers, judges, lawyers, teachers and even social workers (especially in the context of child welfare) provide. This means that while practitioners may participate in case conferences and case planning activities, they are almost never the decision-makers within these processes. As a professional service, child and youth care practice finds itself at the bottom of the hierarchy of public and professional perception within the broader field of human services. This can be frustrating for practitioners, especially given that it is often they who spend the most time with a particular child or youth and who have useful and relevant information and intervention strategies that reflect the child or youth's everyday reality. In fact, one of the most famous books in our field, *The Other 23 Hours*, was written precisely to acknowledge the importance of the practitioner's role in the lifespaces and everyday existence of the child (Trieschman, Whittaker, & Bendtro, 1969).

Equally laden with professional issues are the relationships between child and youth care practitioners, especially in the context of residential care (Ainsworth & Fulcher, 2006; Fulcher, 1991, 2007; Krueger, 1987). Group care also entails group-based responsibilities on the part of the care givers, and here one encounters myriad professional issues that reflect both the best and the worst of the profession. Boundaries between child and youth workers, issues of team loyalty, accountability and transparency, as well as issues of support and guidance all manifest themselves within the relationships between practitioners.

The Context of Self

Arguably one of the most challenging sets of professional issues within child and youth care practice emerges from the exploration of Self (Fewster, 1990; Fewster & Rand, 2001; Garfat, McElwee, & Charles, 2005; Garfat & Charles, 2005). On the one hand, virtually every child and youth care practitioner discovers at some point some of the positive and unexpected strengths and resiliencies that she never knew she had, and this certainly furthers her ability to maintain professional standards and to implement the full complexity of the field on an every day basis. On the other hand, the exploration of Self provides the context in which the identity of the practitioner becomes exposed in relation to children and youth, and here it is not uncommon to be confronted with characteristics and themes that are not always easy to accept. All of the biases, preferences and unsubstantiated beliefs and values of the practitioner suddenly become an integral part of the job, and the professional issues that arise from one's recognition of deficits within one's own identity are virtually endless.

Moreover, it is the professional issues related to the exploration of Self that most obviously cross over to clinical and practice issues as well. It has long been recognized within the field that the Self plays a rather substantive role in how the work with children and youth unfolds, and therefore, it is virtually impossible to separate, even artificially, the professional issues from other issues related to the exploration of Self (Fewster, 1991; Stuart, 2008). And yet, it is equally problematic to discount or omit some consideration of how the Self might impact the professional context and contributions of the child and youth care practitioner. This is where one discovers one's boundaries, one's commitment to confidentiality and the degree to which one is able to abide by the ethical standards of the profession. It is therefore also where any exploration of the professional issues of child and youth care practice ought to start.

PROFESSIONAL ISSUES OF PROFESSIONAL ORGANIZATION

In the series of articles that follows, I have specifically chosen to omit discussion of two sets of professional issues that have had a central place in the literature about the profession itself. One is the issue of whether or not child and youth care practice is in fact a profession and, if so, what its professional characteristics might be. There is a long tradition in this field to discuss and debate the professional status of child and youth care, and contributors have variably concluded that it is indeed a profession (Anglin, 1999; Beker, 2001a), that it is not one (Dunlop, 2004; Jull, 2000), that perhaps it is more of a "craft" (Eisikovits & Beker, 2001), or that it is on its way of becoming a profession (Gaughan & Gharabaghi, 1999). Most of these contributions have in common an approach that involves making a list of characteristics commonly associated with a profession and then comparing that list to what is unfolding in child and youth care practice. A subset of these issues are many contributions in the litera- ture that describe and analyze the degree of professionalization in the field without necessarily committing to whether or not child and youth care practice can be seen as a profession (Beker, 2001b; Berube, 1984; Corney, 2004; Hills, 1989).

In the contemplation of professional issues of child and youth care, it is not terribly important whether or not child and youth care prac- tice is in fact a profession. What matters much more is the substance of the field and what it might mean to the practitioners. What is known is that the field has expanded, offers more opportunity than ever before, and that many practitioners consider it to be their pro- fessional identity. In this sense, then, contemplating the professional issues of child and youth care practice becomes focused on how prac- titioners might make meaning of their experiences as "professionals," rather than whether they can meaningfully compare their endeavor to some predetermined list of criteria that would confirm the pro- fessional status of their discipline.

A second issue, and arguably a much more important one, relates to the organizational infrastructure of the profession. Over the course of the past fifty years, there has been much debate and much activity with respect to the development of professional associations, especially in North America and notably also in South Africa, Scotland, Australia and Israel (Smith, 2002; Stuart, 2001). The motiv- ation behind establishing professional associations relates very much to the issue of professionalizing the discipline, and in many jurisdic- tions, a deep desire to have the discipline recognized through a licens- ing, accreditation or certification process is driving much of the work to organize the profession. The response on the part of practitioners has been limited, and even the largest professional association of child and youth care practitioners in the world can only claim a mem- bership of barely 10% of eligible practitioners (Gharabaghi, 2009).

In reality, a great deal of work needs to be done before the idea of professional organization can take hold in this field. The enormous variations in pre-service qualifications of child and youth care practi- tioners, differences in how and why these practitioners are given job assignments, and uneven levels of commitment to the discipline itself on the part of practitioners continue to challenge the concept of professional organization. Even the name of the profession is uncertain, and there are at least six common titles that are given to child and youth care practitioners in North America alone (child and youth worker, child care worker, child and youth counselor, youth worker, youth development worker, and direct services worker).

On the other hand, there has been some important movement in setting a foundation for professional organization in the field. In North America, the North American Certification project, which aims to set knowledge and skills standards for child and youth workers regardless of setting or job assignment, is one such step. Also relevant is the increasing focus on child and youth care based research and knowledge generation, which has been growing as a result of several university-based departments with an explicit focus on the profession. Even evidence-based practices are emerging within the field and are slowly (and rather unevenly and unreliably) making their way into the practice environments of child and youth workers (Stuart, 2006; 2008).

I have not included a lengthy discussion of professional association simply because of the rapidly changing landscape of this particular aspect of the professional issues in the field. I believe that it is important that we provide a basis for contemplating the core professional issues of the discipline first, make some progress in coming to a common understanding of what child and youth care practitioners are facing in their day-to-day experiences and then begin our focus on professional organization anew. I very much suspect, perhaps optimistically, that the issue of professional organization will warrant its own text in the not so distant future, and certainly that would be a welcome development in our field.

WRITING ABOUT THE PROFESSIONAL ISSUES OF CHILD AND YOUTH CARE

One of the themes that transcends virtually all of the professional issues discussed and contemplated in the series of articles that follows is that of language. By way of an argument, I would suggest that the single greatest professional issue facing child and youth care practitioners everywhere is the relatively low competence (or perhaps interest) in the areas of writing, communication and articulation of conceptual themes. Very much related to this is the sparse engagement of practitioners with the academic or even professional debates that are unfolding in countless journals and professional publications, both in print and online. This creates a significant risk of the development of two quite separate disciplines in child and youth care: one that is "virtual" and exists primarily in the minds of those writing about the discipline, and one that is very real and exists primarily in the actions of those working as child and youth care practitioners every day.

On the one hand, I believe that the tremendous work of academics and professionals who strive to advance the conceptual and theoretical bases of the discipline, and also those who provide us with empirical foundations and evidence bases for what we do, are of great importance and hold the key to a successful future for the discipline as a whole. On the other hand, I also believe that this usefulness is mitigated by the limitations of practitioners in terms of engaging with this material and being able to use this material as the basis for articulating why they do what they do, and for contemplating alternative approaches in their specific work settings.

As a result of this ongoing dilemma between making conceptual contributions to the discipline and wanting these contributions to be of interest to the practitioner, I have chosen a rather eclectic writing style. The goal is to mix theoretical discussion with an engagement of what actually happens in the field in language that ranges from difficult to almost colloquial. It is noteworthy that one of the most accessed sources of information, knowledge and discussion in our field on the part of practitioners is an on-line resource commonly referred to as CYC Net. With approximately 4,000 subscribers, this free internet resource captures most of the core issues of the discipline in formats that range from highly academic to almost conversational and that incorporates multiple language forms seamlessly, including prose, poetry and visual art.

CYC Net provides us with useful lessons in terms of how to engage the field. It presents a bridge between the research and analysis carried out by the many scholars in the field and the day-to-day experiences of the practitioners and, unlike so many other attempts to generate a knowledge sharing environment between these different constituents from within the field, this one actually is characterized by high levels of traffic from all directions. In the spirit of CYC Net, therefore, I have written these articles in a way to be appealing to the thousands of practitioners who are in fact interested in stepping aside from their day-to-day work settings in order to engage in some contemplation, but also in a way that some of the core themes and issues discussed and debated in the academic literature are in fact represented adequately.

The articles that follow are conversational more so than academic but, nevertheless, reflect many different voices in the field. Notably, I have focused my references on academic material that is, in my estimation, particularly accessible to practitioners, such as publications like *Relational Child and Youth Care Practice* and *Reclaiming Youth* and some of the books that were written by significant contributors in the field with the practitioner in mind, including works by Durrant (1993), Maier (1987), Garfat (2003) and Fewster (1991). Of course, this is a discipline with much history, and it is impossible and not desirable in the least to omit some of the voices that gave rise to our field in the first place. Wherever possible, therefore, I have also incorporated references to the works of scholars such as Bronfenbrenner (1979), Bettleheim (1974), and Redl and Wineman (1957), as well as pioneers such as Addams (1910) and Korczak (1925). Presenting the professional issues of child and youth care practice turned out to be a much more complex task than I anticipated; nevertheless, I hope that what follows will capture the imagination of practitioners and the interest of academics alike.

REFERENCES

Addams, J. (1910). *Twenty years at Hull House.* New York: Macmillan.

Anglin, J. (1999). The uniqueness of child and youth care: A personal perspective. *Child and Youth Care Forum, 28*(2), 143–150.

Ainsworth, F., & Fulcher, L. C. (2006). Creating and sustaining a culture of group care. *Child & Youth Services, 28,* 151–176.

Beker, J. (2001a). The emergence of clinical youth work as a profession: Implications for the youth work field. *Child and Youth Care Forum, 30*(6), 373–376.

Beker, J. (2001b). Development of a professional identity for the child care worker. *Child and Youth Care Forum, 30*(6), 345–354.

Berube, P. (1984). Professionalization of child care: A Canadian example. *Journal of Child and Youth Care, 2*(1), 1–12.

Bettelheim, B. (1974). Home for the heart. New York: Knopf.

Bronfenbrenner, U. (1979). *Ecology of human development.* Cambridge, MA: Harvard University Press.

Corney, T. (2004). Values versus competencies: Implications for the future of professional youth work education. *Journal of Youth Studies*, *7*(4), 513–527.

Delano, F. (2001). If I could supervise my supervisor—a model for child and youth care workers to "Own their Own Supervision." *Journal of Child and Youth Care*, *15*(2), 51–64.

Dunlop, T. (2004). Framing a new and expanded vision for the future of child and youth care work: An international, intercultural and trans-disciplinary perspective. *Journal of Child and Youth Care Work*, *19*, 254–267.

Durrant, M. (1993). *Residential treatment: A cooperative, competency-based approach to therapy and program design*. New York: WW Norton & Company.

Eisikovits, Z., & Beker, J. (2001). Beyond professionalism: The child and youth care worker as craftsman. *Child and Youth Care Forum*, *30*(6), 415–434.

Fewster, G. (1982). You, me and us. *Journal of Child Care*, *1*(1), 71–73.

Fewster, G. (1990). *Being in child care: A journey into self*. New York: Haworth Press.

Fewster, G., & Rand, M. (2001). Self, boundaries, and containment: Integrative body psychotherapy. *Journal of Child and Youth Care*, *15*(4), 57–70.

Finlay, J. (2007). *We are your sons and daughters: The Child Advocate's report on the quality of care of 3 Children's Aid Societies*. Toronto, Canada: Office of Child and Family Services Advocacy.

Fulcher, L. (1991). Teamwork in residential care. In J. Beker & Z. Eisikovits (Eds.), *Knowledge utilization in residential child and youth care practice* (pp. 215–235). Washington, DC: Child Welfare League of America.

Fulcher, L. (2007). Residential child and youth care is fundamentally about team work. *Relational Child and Youth Care Practice*, *20*(4), 30–36.

Gannon, B. (2003). Using theory in practice. *CYC OnLine*, *52*(May). Retrieved January 31, 2009, from http://www.cyc-net.org/cyc-online/cycol-0503-theory.html

Garfat, T. (2001). Congruence between supervision and practice. *Journal of Child and Youth Care*, *15*(2), iii–iv.

Garfat, T., & Charles, G. (2005). How am I who I am? Self in child and youth care practice. *Relational Child and Youth Care Practice*, *18*(2), 6–15.

Garfat, T., McElwee, N., & Charles, G. (2005). Self in social care. In S. Share & N. McElwee (Eds.), *Applied social care: An introduction for Irish students* (pp. 112–120). Dublin: Gill and McMillan.

Gaughan, P., & Gharabaghi, K. (1999). The prospects and dilemmas of child and youth work as a professional discipline. *Journal of Child and Youth Care*, *13*(1), 1–18.

Gharabaghi, K. (2005). Promoting organizational change in response to the YCJA. In A. Lockhart & L. Zammit (Eds.), *Restorative justice: Transforming society* (pp. 122–125). Toronto, Canada: Inclusion Press.

Gharabaghi, K. (2009). Organizing the profession. *CYC OnLine*, *120*(February). Retrieved February 1, 2009, from http://www.cyc-net.org/cyc-online/cyconline-feb2009-gharabaghi.html

Hills, M. D. (1989). The child and youth care student as an emerging professional practitioner. *Journal of Child and Youth Care*, *4*(1), 17–31.

Jull, D. (2000). Is child and youth care a profession? *Journal of Child and Youth Care*, *14*(3), 79–88.

Ingram, G., & Harris, J. (2001). *Delivering good youth work: A working guide to thriving and surviving*. Dorset, UK: Russell House Publishing.

Korczak, J. (1992). *When I am little again and the child's right to respect*. New York: University Press of America.

Krueger, M. (1987). Making the team approach work in residential group care. *Child Welfare, 66*, 447–457.

Magnuson, D., & Burger, L. (2001). Developmental supervision in residential care. *Journal of Child and Youth Care, 15*(1), 9–22.

Maier, H. (1985). Teaching and training as a facet of supervision of child care staff: An overview. *Journal of Child Care, 2*(4), 49–52.

Maier, H. (2003). What to say when first meeting a person each day. *Relational Child and Youth Care Practice, 16*(3), 40–41.

Mann-Feder, V. (2001). The self as subject in child and youth care supervision. *Journal of Child and Youth Care, 15*(2), 1–8.

Moore, P. (2001). Critical components of an anti-oppressive framework. *Journal of Child and Youth Care, 14*(3), 25–32.

Phelan, J. (1990). Child care supervision: The neglected skill of evaluation. In J. P. Anglin, C. J. Denhom, R. V. Ferguson, & A. R. Pence (Eds.), *Perspectives in professional child and youth care* (pp. 182–194). New York: Haworth.

Phelan, J. (2000). To each his own: Theory and practice models. *CYC OnLine, 22*(December). Retrieved January 31, 2009, from http://www.cyc-net.org/cyc-online/cycol-1200-phelan.html

Phelan, J. (2008, October). *Child and youth care is complex!* Paper presented at the meeting of the Canadian National Child and Youth Care Conference, Charlottetown, PEI.

Ragg, M., Patrick, D., & Ziefert, M. (2006). Slamming the closet door: Working with gay and lesbian youth in care. *Child Welfare, 85*(2), 243–265.

Redl, F., & Wineman, D. (1957). *The aggressive child*. Glencoe, IL: Free Press.

Ricks, F. (1989). Self-awareness model for training and application in child and youth care. *Journal of Child and Youth Care, 4*(1), 33–41.

Schissel, B. (1997). *Blaming children: Youth crime, moral panics and the politics of hate*. Halifax, NS: Fernwood Publishing.

Skott-Myhre, H. (2006). Radical youth work: Becoming visible. *Child and Youth Care Forum, 35*(3), 219–229.

Smith, M. (2002). Stands Scotland where it did? Perspectives and possibilities for child and youth care. *CYC On-Line, 47*. Retrieved December 22, 2008 from www.cyc-net.org/cyc-online/cyccol-1202-smith-scotland.html

Stuart, C. (2001). Professionalizing child and youth care: Continuing the Canadian journey. *Journal of Child and Youth Care Work, 16*, 264–282.

Stuart, C. (2008). Editorial: Theory, research and praxis. *Relational Child and Youth Care Practice, 21*(1), 3–6.

Trieschman, A. E., Whittaker, A., & Bendtro, L. (1969). *The other 23 hours: Child care work with emotionally disturbed children in a therapeutic milieu*. New York: Aldine de Gruyter.

VanderVen, K. (2003). Transforming the milieu and lives through the power of activity: Theory and practice. *Journal of Child and Youth Care Work*, *19*, 103–108.

Weisman, V. (1999). Relationships: What is it we do? . . . It is what we do! *Journal of Child and Youth Care*, *13*(2), 125–131.

Winfield, J. (2005). Thinking theory, doing practice. *Child and Youth Care*, *23*(8), 22–23.

Boundaries and the Exploration of Self

SUMMARY. Boundaries and the exploration of self are conceptualized within the agency-structure problem first articulated in social theory during the 1970s. Constructing boundaries as a professional issue within the discipline has to take account the agency embedded within boundaries. Multiple boundary dilemmas are discussed within the framework of the agency-structure problem, including those that result from policies and procedures, and it is further argued that boundaries and the exploration of self also impact at the team level. Finally, the role of power imbalances within the practice of boundary formation is explored in relational worker–client interactions.

KEYWORDS. Boundaries, exploration of Self, agency and structure, professional issues in child and youth care practice, team work

It is surprisingly challenging to explore the *professional issues* related to boundaries and the exploration of Self. In our profession, managing the Self and constructing boundaries lie at the core of everything we do, and the implications for doing so cannot be neatly separated into a set of professional issues and sets of other kinds of issues (Ingram & Harris, 2001; Krueger, 2004,

2007). Sometimes constructing boundaries is the intervention we might use as a core element of a treatment plan; other times, boundaries are constructed as a way of defining our professional identity within a particular practice setting (Garfat, 1993). In theory, boundaries and the exploration of Self are the foundation of child and youth care practice and permeate all relationships we encounter in our work. We cannot separate boundaries and the exploration of Self precisely because these two concepts are inter-dependent. Boundaries are constructed *through* the exploration of Self (Buffie, 2004; Fewster, 2004; Garfat, 1999). In practice, on the other hand, the construction of boundaries is impacted as much by our identity as practitioners as it is impacted by the organizational culture within which we work and by the policies and procedures imposed by the institution or the employer. In this article, I will explore specifically the boundaries of Self inasmuch as these relate to how the practitioner frames his interactions and co-presence with others, including clients and other professionals. I will not specifically explore the boundaries of professional responsi-bility. However, at least to some extent, professional boundaries in any context pertain to the extent and scope of professional responsi-bility as well.

Given the challenges associated with the discussion of boundaries and the exploration of Self as professional issues distinct from clinical or other types of issues, it is necessary to provide some artificial struc-ture for the task at hand. This is necessary in order to ensure that we remain conscious of the interconnectedness of all things within our discipline. And still, I hope that we can impose this structure as a way of exploring issues and themes in a manner that highlights these without severing them from the living and organic work that we do.

Let us start with a number of assumptions about the exploration of Self, as it pertains to the practitioner. First, let us assume that "explo-ration" implies process. Specifically, it implies a multi-dimensional process rather than a linear process. When we explore, we are not simply stepping from one rest stop to the next on the road to a well defined destination. Exploration requires that we step out into all directions, forward and backwards, up and down, and that we seek out experiences through a continuous reshuffling of variables, issues, activities, themes, and choices and decisions. In exploring we seek to experience and make meaning, not to arrive at and conquer a desti-nation or a difficult path. As Krueger (2007, p. 40) put it, "The goal is to be *in* development *with* youth and to constantly seek ways to learn and grow while experiencing the moment and/or the activity together."

We will assume, moreover, that the Self which we are exploring is itself not a closed system or entity. By this I mean that we are not thinking about the Self as a space with defined dimensions, such as a box or a cave or a house. Instead, we understand that the Self is itself changing and evolving on a continuous basis. The changes reflect new information, new influences, new experiences and new meanings absorbed through the passage of time and the Self's exposure and connection to all things in the physical, intellectual and metaphorical environments surrounding it. The exploration of the Self, therefore, is a process that does not—that cannot—lead to an end; it is a life long journey that at best can produce moments of clarity and self-assuredness. Again, according to Krueger (2007, p. 41), "... youth workers view life as a process of human interaction in which meaning is conferred to any situation by the perspectives people bring to it from their subjective value systems ... new meanings are made each time a person interacts with another person in a specific context or situation and these meanings become part of their evolving narratives."

Our third assumption is perhaps the most complex one. The exploration of Self does not ask the question "who am I?" Instead, it asks the question "how shall I constitute my Self right now?" We might alternatively phrase the question as "how is my Self constituted right now?" but if we do so, we change the meaning of exploring our Self considerably. This second phrasing of the question implies passivity and a lack of choice. The Self is constituted by something other or in response to something other. In contrast, the first question allows for choice and agency. The assumption of agency is a critical one. Without it, we become objects in our work shaped by our connections to children, institutions, rules and norms, and ethics. Moreover, without an assumption of agency, child and youth workers are denied their individuality, their uniqueness as individuals, and their role in shaping, fostering or fighting that uniqueness. By allowing for agency, in contrast, child and youth workers become subjects to their thoughts and actions, and each child and youth worker has the privilege and the responsibility of constituting a Self fit for the moment.

Still working with this third assumption, we do have to qualify our agency; while there is choice there is also structure. By structure I mean all of those elements impacting our Self in ways that we cannot control. Structure in this sense can mean policies and procedures or it can mean aspects of our identity that are present as constants such as our gender, our culture, our race, and our religion. Of course, none of these elements of identity are set in stone either. How we make meaning of our gender, our race, or any of the other identity elements reflects our agency. There is, therefore, a degree of elasticity in this structure that is activated by our agency while, at the same time, the degree of choice within agency is impacted considerably by the structure. This is known as the agent-structure problem in social theory. Does structure shape agency or does agency shape structure?

This question has long been subject to debate within the literature of social theory. Structuralists argue that structure shapes agency, while reductionists contend that agency shapes structure (Dosse, 1997; Rosenberg, 2007; Sturrock, 2003). For our purposes, we will accept a theoretical re-construction of this problem first articulated by the British sociologist Anthony Giddens (1977; 1979). Giddens provided us with the foundation for structuration theory, and its central premise that agency and structure are interdependent and are locked in a perpetual process of mutual shaping. We can readily identify parallels for this in some of the child and youth care literature, even if such parallels are not articulated within the context of structuration theory. Krueger's metaphor of child and youth care as a "dance" suggests a similar relationship between agency and structure (Krueger, 2004). While the dancers choose their steps and carefully manage their physical responses to each other and to the music, the music provides the structure for their movements and directs them as they glide across the floor. And yet each dancing couple moves slightly differently, making choices as they dance and producing their own unique way of being within the musical structure.

So far, we have only discussed the exploration of Self, and we have articulated some assumptions we make about that process. As child and youth workers, we do not simply explore our Self for fun; we do so as a way of making meaning of our experiences with children, families and communities, and we use that meaning to guide us in our actions and our decisions about how to be in the presence of others. It is here where we find the connection between our Self, however constituted, and the concept of boundaries.

It is important to articulate from the outset the most critical differences between boundaries in our discipline and boundaries as they might exist elsewhere. A boundary is fundamentally a static concept, one that is constructed in a place where it is to protect what is inside of it from that which might intrude. Boundaries have an impact by virtue of their presence; they are not typically seen as "active" entities. Boundaries don't *do* anything. Within our discipline, however, boundaries are not static at all, and they serve much more than a protective function. Boundaries in child and youth care are active in the sense that they reach out to the other in order to construct very specific types of connections. Within our discipline, boundaries are relational and act as the ambassadors for our Self. Boundaries give something to the other, and they are constructed not as a spatial concept but as a communicative and engaging concept. In contrast to child and youth care practice, in other disciplines, and notably in mainstream social work, the connection of boundaries and Self has often been severed (Mandell, 2008).

Much like we had to make some assumption about the process of exploring our Self, we now have to make some assumptions about the process of constructing boundaries. Let us start with reiterating the previous point. Boundaries are the ambassadors for our Self. They express to the other what at this moment represents the constitution of our Self. They transcend the separation of our Self from the Self of the other. Without boundaries, exploring our Self becomes a self-serving (but still valuable) project with little to offer to the other. In this sense, boundaries are what make our profession a relational one.

A second assumption that is necessary is that boundaries change in relation to changes to the Self, not in relation to whoever the other might be. In fact, boundaries are not responsive to the other but rather to the Self. This seems quite logical given the previous discussions, but it is counterintuitive given our day-to-day practice. It would seem much more logical to change one's boundaries based on who we are dealing with in the moment. We might construct one set of boundaries for colleagues, another for supervisors, and yet another for the children or youth we work with. But we do not. Instead, we construct our boundaries in response to the exploration of Self which, as we discussed earlier, is influenced as much by the structural context in which we are present as it is influenced by our own choices and decisions.

So long as we conceptualize boundaries as the ambassador for our Self rather than as the response to the other, we maintain an integrity for our actions that exempts the other from baring responsibility for broken connections. This forces us to understand relationships as manifestations of relational activity rather than as outcomes of coexistence. The boundaries we impose on the other reflect the status of our exploration of Self, negotiated within the ongoing agent-structure problem, and these boundaries reflect the extension of our exploration onto the other. Where boundaries reflect co-existence, there is not relational activity; only where boundaries reflect exploration of Self can relational activity emerge.

Let us now summarize some of the core assumptions based on which we will examine the exploration of Self and the construction of boundaries as professional issues:

- The exploration of Self is a process that will never end;
- This process is influenced by structure but the structure is also shaped by the choices we make;
- Boundaries are constructed in relation to the exploration of Self;
- Boundaries are the ambassadors of the Self;
- Boundaries are never static but, instead, they reflect our relational engagement with the other.

STRUCTURE AND AGENCY IN THE EXPLORATION OF SELF

The exploration of Self takes place within an elastic structure of identity elements that we cannot change but to which we can give meaning based on our own experiences and interpretations. Some of these elements can readily be identified: gender, race, ethnicity, sexual orientation, physical disability, mental capacity, and so on. Our experience with respect to each of these identity elements is shaped to some degree by the socially constructed meanings associated with each element. There is no denying that one's gender, for example, cannot escape the social roles, stereotypes, and expectations imposed by the broader articulations of gender politics. Similarly, one's ethnicity contributes to the exploration of Self at the structural level based on the much broader societal expectations and assumptions about specific ethnic groups.

Some identity elements impact on the construction of Self from birth; much research has been done to demonstrate the influences of gender politics on the socialization process of very young children.

Indeed, choosing pink for a girl and blue for a boy even before the child is born clearly indicates just how much we are shaped by structural impositions on identity formation. Other identity elements may provide structural impositions much later in the developmental process. Sexual orientation or questioning, for example, does not typically manifest itself until the pre-teen or even teenage years, and therefore, the construction of Self becomes subject to the structural influence of sexual politics a little later. Some elements of identity may be subject to structural shaping on an intermittent basis. This is the case especially for those identity elements that move from the periphery to the centre of political discourse based on world events and movement within political culture. Ethnicity, for example, might not have been a core element of identity until the world shifted its focus on the war on terrorism. Suddenly being of Middle Eastern ethnicity might well become a core element of identity for some, displacing previous core elements unrelated to current world events.

The structural elements associated with identity formation shape our exploration of Self within the public realm. All of these elements have histories and linguistic conventions that are generated from their exposure within that public realm. But structural elements within the exploration of Self are not limited to the public realm; they also appear in the private realm, often with equal or even greater consequence.

All of us have histories that reflect our unique experiences from birth to the present day. Who we are is very much shaped by where we came from. In this sense, our family experiences, our connections within family, neighborhoods and communities and the customs and conventions embedded within these all serve as structural elements impacting our exploration of Self. We cannot fully disassociate ourselves from this history. Specific experiences within our private realms may manifest themselves at very high levels of consciousness for long periods of time. Such experiences, therefore, may have shaping influences within our exploration of Self. The experience of abuse, for example, may well create a dominant reflective filter within the exploration of Self that channels the explorative process toward a singular or unidimensional view of identity and Self. For some, the absence of defining moments in their history within the private realm may allow for an unlimited or unrestricted process of exploration, shaped still by structural elements but not channeled towards a singular theme or experience acting as a reflective filter.

The point is that it is important to remain conscious of the influences of broader social movements and their resultant political discourse in the exploration of the Self. Similarly, it is critical to evaluate the structural elements of the private realm as well. Our private experiences have structural characteristics to the extent that they shape our exploration of Self. On the other hand, it is equally important to remember that we do not have universal responses to these influences. In fact, our agency in the exploration of Self very much impacts the degree to which we counter the structural shaping of identity and Self. In giving meaning to the broader social and political discourse surrounding questions of identity, we make choices. And in making these choices, we are shaping the structural elements while being shaped by them. This brings us back to structuration theory, where agency and structure are locked in a perpetual process of mutual shaping. And it also brings us back to the topic of boundaries, since the relationship between the exploration of Self and the construction of boundaries very much mirrors the dynamics of structure and agency respectively.

BOUNDARIES AS AGENCY

Every child and youth care practitioner has had to grapple with boundaries well before they joined the profession. After all, everyone continuously applies boundaries in personal relationships, and everyone makes decisions about self-disclosure, touch and relationships within their family, their neighborhood, and their community. As child and youth care practitioners, however, we are confronted with a unique situation in which to make decisions about boundaries. In addition to maintaining the rationales for our boundary decisions outside of our professional role, we now must integrate that professional role into our private existence. This may not be entirely obvious, and therefore it may require some explanation.

On the surface, it ought to be possible to step out of our private lives and temporarily assume our professional role as a distinct role that is entirely separate from our private existence. We do know, after all, precisely when we take on our professional role (at the start of a shift or at the moment of encounter with a client) and when we cease to fulfill that role (at the end of the shift or after saying good bye to the client for the day). So why should it not be possible to simply leave our personal Self behind and to adopt our professional Self once we are on the job?

This is where the nature of child and youth care practice differs substantially from other professions, including other helping professions. Child and Youth Care work takes place within the life spaces of children, youth and families and, as such, our professional activities unfold within our clients' private lives. Moreover, the goals of our profession, while diverse and multi-faceted, never include the goal of imposing change on the life space of the client, nor of imposing such change on the client. While change is a hoped-for outcome of our interventions/presence, the kind of change we are aiming to foster is not directed at either the environment or the client, but rather at the manner in which the client relates to his or her life spaces. We might hope for greater adaptive functioning, or we might hope for greater resilience on the part of the client, but we do not typically arrive at the client's life space with a blueprint for change. Instead, we offer our presence, sometimes passively and sometimes in active and engaging ways, as a way of providing a relational opportunity for the client to reconstitute his Self through new experiences, remodeled memories of past experiences, and reconstituted aspirations and expectations for the future.

Unlike an engineer who offers her client a structural blueprint for a bridge, or an accountant who offers his client a spreadsheet for financial matters, we offer our client us. And unlike a psychologist who offers her client an explanation or a social worker who might offer a client a solution to a problem, our presence offers an experience of being: with someone, in spite of someone, connected and related.

In offering ourselves, we expose our Self, whether we intend to do so or not. In encouraging relatedness, connections, relationships, we must present in a transparent and accessible manner. And we must be flexible enough to allow the client to find his or her connection to us. We cannot simply present a "professional identity" that the client can take or leave. And we must be responsive and reciprocate the connection. Without that responsiveness, our presence would be reduced to an outlet for the client to "plug into."

Exposing our Self is no easy task. For one thing, we are still exploring our Self and we are almost certainly uncertain about where this exploration will take us next. Moreover, our exploration will be impacted by this new relationship, these new circumstances we are encountering by being with the client. Essentially, we have placed ourselves in a situation where our exploration of Self unfolds parallel to the client's exploration of Self, and we are consciously creating moments where these two exploration processes intersect and join together. To maintain a sense of personal safety and to protect the integrity of our exploration of Self, we create boundaries that fit the circumstances and respond to the needs of our Self.

It is in this sense that the relationship between the Self and boundaries mirrors the relationship between structure and agency. The Self serves as the structural element influencing our articulation of boundaries, while the boundaries reflect our choices with respect to how much we are prepared to expose the Self. At the same time, the choices we make about boundaries impact the exploration of Self, and therefore shape the structure represented by the Self as much as that structure is shaping the agency represented by the boundaries we have created.

When we are able to recognize our boundaries as an expression of agency, we are also able to acknowledge that our boundaries are not reflective of who we are but, rather, of where we are in our process of exploration of Self. And this provides us with an opportunity to fuel our exploration of Self in new and exciting ways, because what is at stake is not our identity (who we are) but the direction our exploration will follow next (where we will go). And if we can assist our client in understanding his boundaries as agency in the process of exploring *his* Self, then our work becomes a joint exploration of Self through the agencies of our boundaries.

In the next section of this article, we will focus on the much more practical issues of specific boundary choices, and we will try to relate these back to the theoretical framework for the exploration of Self and boundaries explored above.

PRACTICE DILEMMAS IMPACTING SELF AND BOUNDARIES

It is an unfortunate fact of life that child and youth care practice unfolds not only within the context of doing the best we can for the client, but also within an employment context. Someone hires us to do what we do, and by virtue of being the employer, that someone has the right and obligation to set the parameters within which we will have to work. Such parameters account for a very broad range of issues and themes, and typically include at least the following:

- Employment expectations about when we work, how many hours per week, when we start each day and when we finish;
- Policies and procedures defining how we work, what practices are acceptable or unacceptable, and what outcomes are expected of us;
- Safety procedures outlining requirements for interacting with clients, what spaces are safe or not safe, what interventions might be required in certain situations;
- Reporting requirements detailing what we must record, what information we must share, when we must report, and to whom we must report.

From the perspective of the employer, these kinds of rules and regulations are indispensable, frequently required by law, and almost always designed to ensure that the work of many people from multiple disciplines unfolds smoothly, predictably, meaningfully and maintains whatever standards the employer might be aiming for. In addition, some of these rules and regulations are in place to manage resources, including financial resources, to manage risk, and to contain liabilities for the worker and for the organization. While the necessity of having to manage resources, risk and liabilities might be lamentable, it certainly would not be wise to abstain from managing these items. On the other hand, having predetermined rules and regulations about how, when and with whom we do our work presents us with some significant practice dilemmas that can reasonably be described as professional issues within our discipline.

The Policy and Procedures Manual

Policy and Procedures Manuals have a number of characteristics that can potentially create some significant dilemmas for child and youth workers. First and foremost, these manuals create the rules by which we have to abide, and these rules are typically articulated as having universal applicability. Therein lays our first dilemma. Our clients are not all the same, their circumstances differ substantially, and their capacity to follow or be guided by one predetermined approach to service is likely limited. This presents a major challenge to child and youth care practitioners, who hold as one of their core values the recognition of difference and uniqueness of each and every client. Working in the life spaces of children, youth and families by definition requires openness to a very broad range of possibilities.

To the extent that the policy and procedures manual spells out some direction about "professional" boundaries, we encounter our first challenge to the child and youth care framework for thinking about boundaries. As we discussed earlier in this article, boundaries provide agency within our exploration of Self, and therefore the specific nature of boundaries that we, as individual child and youth care practitioners, might want to explore may or may not correspond to the definition or description of professional boundaries as outlined in the manual. We will discuss this further below, but for now, I want to emphasize the challenges associated with having a document of universal applicability govern the work of a discipline that holds individualization and customization of service as a core value (Ingram & Harris, 2001).

We encounter a similar challenge in the context of operationalizing the child and youth care concept of "experiencing." Within our discipline, the importance of making meaning through an experiential process as opposed to an explanatory process is well established (Richmond, 2006; Stuart, 2008). The policy framework typically contained in a manual, on the other hand, speaks to timelines, reporting requirements and safety considerations that significantly undermine the possibility of experiencing, either on the part of the client or on the part of the child and youth workers.

Perhaps the most notable dilemma with respect to the policy and procedures manual is the incongruence between the language of the manual versus that of our profession. Indeed, the very conceptualization of what constitutes professional conduct differs substantially between the manual and our practice. In most cases written by administrators rather than practitioners, policy and procedures manuals provide a framework for professional conduct that assumes a separation of professional identity and personal identity, of the public realm and the private realm. This, as we discussed earlier, is highly problematic for our profession, in which the concept of "professional" includes deeply entrenched roles for secondary concepts such as informality, spontaneity, relational engagement, and interpersonal relationships. It is nearly impossible to merge the language of policy and procedures with the language of caring and engagement as it is reflected in our profession.

Policy-Driven Boundaries

It is enormously difficult to "do" child and youth work if we cannot constitute our boundaries in response to our exploration of Self. Working with boundaries that feel wrong, uncomfortable, or foreign to us creates a weak and vulnerable foundation for relational engagement with children, youth, or families. It also severs agency from structure in that an imposed approach to boundary formation will fail to shape our exploration of Self and be shaped by that exploration. In this sense, it creates disequilibrium in the perpetual process of mutual shaping discussed earlier.

And yet as practitioners within a defined employment context, we are constantly challenged in terms of boundaries. In many practice settings, policies pursuant to appropriate boundaries abound. Thus we find articulations of "no touch" policies, rules about where we take clients, who we introduce them to and when we engage with them. We also find policies about self disclosure, gift giving and receiving and confidentiality. All of these rules and policies serve important purposes from the perspective of the employer, and we should not simply dismiss them as ill-conceived or reflective of bad thinking. On the other hand, these rules and policies typically reflect priorities that do not fit very well with ours. While no touch policies may well reduce the risk of allegations, law suits and lengthy complaint processes, from our perspective, these policies also de-humanize our work with children and violate our commitment to a developmental approach to caring for children (Smith, 2004; 2006). Similarly, while rules about self-disclosure might well reduce the chances of disorder and discord in staff–client relationships, not having the flexibility to share with a child, a youth or a family, elements of one's own Self seriously undermines the nature of relational engagement that is feasible. Indeed, it is quite clear that very rigid approaches to self disclosure are reflective of the priorities of other disciplines (notably psychoanalysis and counseling psychology) rather than of any principles of child and youth care. This is not to suggest that unmitigated self disclosure is necessary or even useful in the context of relational child and youth care; it is, however, one of many possible scenarios that might complement a relational approach in specific circumstances, particularly where it reflects, or gives agency to, the exploration of Self undertaken by the child and youth worker.

One of the core professional issues we face as practitioners with respect to the exploration of Self and boundaries is the separation of how we conceive of these themes in theory and how we manage these themes in practice. In theory, everything that we have discussed so far really pertains to a segregated and unreal scenario. We are imagining ourselves face-to-face with a client but in the absence of any particular context. By context I mean both the employment context we have explored above, but also the human context of working in teams, with multiple disciplines and through the involvement of multiple sectors, organizations and interests. In practice, we do not typically have the opportunity to simply sideline these contexts and allow ourselves to be only with the client. The exploration of Self and its resultant boundaries are influenced very strongly by these contexts.

Employers typically are not asking of us to be "ourselves" or even to explore our Self. They are asking us to represent the organization with a professional identity that reflects the organization's values and its mission and mandate. The pressure to conform in spite of our Self is often significant, and the consequences of deviating from the expectations can be severe. We find that even where organizations are supportive of the process of exploring Self, and have some understanding of its importance, there is still a human context that is much more difficult to contain. Most child and youth care unfolds within a team context, and group expectations about how to conduct oneself are usually articulated strongly and imposingly. In residential care settings, themes and concepts such as consistency, order, control and behavior management frequently are priorities, and the team requires conformity with an informal notion of "team Self."

As practitioners, therefore, we are not typically able to make decisions about issues such as self disclosure or physical touch reflecting solely our exploration of Self; we do have to take into consideration the broader context of group dynamics, team expectations, and employer requirements. Programs that operate with no touch policies, for example, are not usually open to child and youth care practitioners who break those policies because of whatever stage they might have reached in their exploration of Self.

Given these limitations of our practice context, it is important to contemplate some of the different ways in which we can maintain the integrity of exploring Self and articulating boundaries as agency of this process while at the same time remaining conscious of the requirement to conform to outside notions of professional identity. In other words, we cannot translate our exploration of Self into actions related to boundaries directly; in most cases, we must first articulate the rationale for this process, advocate on behalf of the discipline, and assist with the exploration of the notion of "team Self."

EXPLORING TEAM SELF

The concept of Self subsumes the concept of identity, but it is not synonymous to identity. We might think of the concept of identity as much more static than the concept of Self, in the sense that identity refers to a set of characteristics or attributes that might be seen as being of consequence to how a person sees himself. Within the discourse about identity, there is recognition of shifting priorities in terms of specific characteristics or attributes based on circumstances and broader ecological developments, but identity remains a descriptive concept with no life of its own. It is the Self that gives it life and that pushes identity into agency.

The Self subsumes identity, but it also provides us with a framework for responding to our identity in a social context. It is through the Self that we merge our complex and internal experiences of emotional, physical, spiritual and ethical sensations. And it is through the Self that we present ourselves in relational engagements and relationships with other. As such, it is fair to say that the concept of Self is one typically associated with the individual, not with groups or teams.

On the other hand, much of what we actually do day in and day out does unfold within the context of teams, and the characteristics of a team are much more than the sum of each of its members' Selves. Teams very much take on a life of their own, and the characteristics of that life cannot adequately be captured through a description of the team's identity (Krueger, 2004). We might be able to identify a team based on many different identity variables but, in and of itself, this does not give us a good understanding about how that team functions. In fact, often times, it gives us a strong misunderstanding about how teams function. We might, for example, identify a team as being experienced, because each member of the team has been working in the field for quite some time or perhaps because the members of the team have been together on that team for some time. This may well be an accurate description of the team, but it tells us nothing at all about how that team functions. The description of experience as a function of time does not imply effectiveness, nor does it imply knowledge or skill (Flint, 1966). A team that has been ineffective for a long period of time would also be described as experienced within these parameters of the definition or description. Alternatively, we might describe a team as being diverse, because the membership of the team includes individuals of varying cultural backgrounds. Again, this may well be accurate, but it tells us nothing about the team's cultural competence or its effectiveness with respect to a diverse group of clients. The mere presence of difference bears no consequence to the knowledge and understanding of diversity and its implications.

In order to really understand a team, we must explore its notion of Self, much like we are obliged to do individually. The team Self is constituted similarly as the individual Self, and team actions are reflections of that Self much like individual actions reflect the process of exploring Self on the part of the individual child and youth care practitioner. There are, however, also differences in the way teams constitute their Self compared to how an individual practitioner might do so, and these are worthy of some consideration (Bettleheim, 1974; Durrant, 1993; Krueger, 1986).

Much like identity is subsumed by the exploration of Self, so teams subsume the dynamics of the group. Group dynamics have long been subject to study in many different fields, and one notable conclusion drawn about group dynamics is that this dynamic tends to reduce the functional and emotional intelligence of the individual group member. In one of his rare mentions of groups, Sigmund Freud went as far as suggesting that groups render its members "stupid" (Freud, 1920). This observation runs somewhat counter to considerations of teams within child and youth care, and especially within residential child and youth care practice. We typically see teams as having a positive impact on working with children and youth. This is the case because teams provide for the opportunity of greater accountability (child and youth workers questioning or critically evaluating each others' actions), an opportunity to vent and seek support from one another (thereby mitigating the risk of burnout), and an opportunity to expose children and youth to a range of valuable relationships. All of this is true and reasonably reflects one reality of teams. There is, however, another reality to be considered. Teams are also characterized by internal loyalty (which can pit child and youth worker against children on behalf of teammates), informal authority processes, informal leadership, and demands for conformity and rule abidance.

Many teams develop their concept of Self through an uneven and typically undemocratic process of creating team cultures. Such cultures are based on values and norms with respect to control, authority, boundaries, commitment, work ethic and team inclusivity. This broad set of categories and themes become molded into one package and reflects a particular and often very rigid expression of team culture. This is often further exacerbated by team positions with respect to management and employment expectation that can range from collaborative and accommodating to resistant and dishonest.

It is important for the practitioner to be aware of this context of his exploration of Self. Wherever that exploration may take him, the reality is that his Self is not the only Self that will determine his actions or his positions with respect to children and youth. The team Self exerts a powerful influence on the practitioner, sometimes for the better, but often for the worse. At a minimum, the team Self mitigates the degree to which the practitioner can claim ownership of the process of exploring his Self.

POWER, BOUNDARIES, AND THE EXPLORATION OF SELF

So far in this article, we have spent considerable time examining both theoretical and practical elements of exploring the Self and giving agency to the Self through the constitution of boundaries. In order to conclude this article, it is necessary to take some time to expose these concepts to the often covert interventions of the concept of power.

Child and youth care as a discipline and a practice cannot avoid the centrality of power within its discourse and practice (Batsleer, 2008). Power is a very complex concept. As an action concept, power can be defined as the ability to influence someone to do something they might not otherwise do. The tools of power might include force, but within our discipline it more commonly includes authority, access to information and physical resources, and persuasion. Power is much more than an action concept; it impacts significantly on how one constitutes one's Self. Power is frequently bestowed not by specific actions, but rather by positions, contexts and information (Ingram & Harris, 2002).

In order to remain conscious of the power imbalances we maintain between ourselves and our clients, it is helpful to list the many ways in which clients might experience our presence as disempowering:

- Our clients depend on child and youth workers for being cared for;
- Our clients have less information than the child and youth workers;
- Our clients have less access to physical spaces than do the child and youth workers;
- Our clients are more monitored and supervised than the child and youth workers;
- Our clients have fewer escape routes than do child and youth workers;
- In a team context, child and youth workers have team resources, whereas clients cannot draw on such resources.

This list could certainly be expanded, perhaps limitlessly. We do have to consider the implications of these power imbalances (Dean, Harpe, & Mallett, 2008; Tompkins-Rosenblatt, 2004). Once again, while the ideal model of the exploration of Self and the constituting of boundaries is based on one child and youth worker face to face and on a relatively even plane with one client, in reality, this is hardly the case. Our exploration of Self and the resultant constitution of boundaries is taking place in the presence of clients who are significantly disempowered within their ecological context. This results in some very practical professional issues to be considered with respect to boundaries in particular. As Batsleer (2008, p. 105) puts it, "Adult/child relationships are caught within a matrix of power, in which many aspects of identity, particularly in this context perhaps dynamics of gender and sexuality, create the context for developing ethical practice."

If we think about self disclosure, for example, and its connection to our exploration of Self, we can readily identify that while we make decisions about the nature and degree of self disclosure, and while we maintain the right to avoid self disclosure, we do not extend the same right to our clients. In fact, in most practice settings, the very processes of getting to know the client relies on the client's preparedness to self disclose, regardless of whether or not she really wants to or is ready to given her exploration of Self.

It is therefore quite critical to remain aware that our exploration of Self is, amongst other things, also a way of wielding power amongst the disempowered. And our constituting of boundaries reflects the disempowerment of the clients while concomitantly perpetuating the power imbalance between ourselves and the clients. We have thus come full circle in our discussion of the *professional issues* entailed in the exploration of Self and the constituting of boundaries. We argued at the beginning of the article that it is not really possible to fully separate professional issues from other kinds of issues. Somewhere and somehow, our professional issues will impact the experience of the client, and whether we refer to this as a clinical issue or simply as a relational issue in no way changes the reality that like all professional issues, the exploration of Self shapes our actions as much as it is shaped by those actions.

REFERENCES

Batsleer, J. R. (2008). *Informal learning in youth work*. London: SAGE.

Bettleheim, B. (1974). *A home for the heart*. New York: Alfred A. Knopf.

Buffie, J. B. (2004). Knowing boundaries. *Relational Child and Youth Care Practice, 17*(1), 51–53.

Dean, M., Harpe, M., Lee, C., & Mallett, A. (2008). Making the familiar strange: Deconstructing developmental psychology in child and youth care. *Relational Child & Youth Care Practice, 21*(3), 43–56.

Dosse, F. (1997). *History of structuralism*. Minneapolis. MN: University of Minnesota Press.

Durrant, M. (1993). *Residential treatment: A cooperative, competency-based approach to therapy and program design*. New York: Norton & Company.

Fewster, G. (2004). Just between you and me: Personal boundaries in professional relationships. *Relational Child and Youth Care Practice, 17*(3), 8–17.

Flint, B. M. (1966). *The child and the institution: A study of deprivation and recovery*. Toronto: University of Toronto Press.

Freud, S. (1920). *Group psychology and the analysis of the ego*. New York: Boni and Liveright.

Garfat, T. (1993). Never alone: Reflections on the presence of self and history in child and youth care work. *Journal of Child and Youth Care Work, 9,* 35–43.

Garfat, T. (1999). Editorial: Questions about self and relationship. *Journal of Child and Youth Care, 13*(2), iii–iv.

Giddens, A. (1977). *Studies in social and political theory*. London: Hutchinson.

Giddens, A. (1979). *Central problems in social theory: Action, structure and contradiction in social analysis*. Berkeley, CA: University of California Press.

Ingram, G., & Harris, J. (2001). *Delivering good youth work: A working guide to thriving and surviving*. Dorset, UK: Russell House Publishing.

Krueger, M. (1986). *Job satisfaction for child and youth workers*. Washington, DC: Child Welfare League of America.

Krueger, M. (2004). *Themes and stories in youth work practice*. New York: The Haworth Press.

Krueger, M. (2007). *Sketching youth, self, and youth work*. Rotterdam: Sense Publishers.

Mandell, D. (2008). Power, care and vulnerability: Considering use of self in child welfare work. *Journal of Social Work Practice, 22*(2), 235–248.

Richmond, P. A. (2006). Boundary realities from the wisdom of female youth in residential treatment. *Journal of Child and Youth Care Work, 21*, 80–93.

Rosenberg, A. (2007). *Philosophy of social science*. Boulder, CO: Westview Press.

Smith, M. (2004). Limiting liability. *CYC OnLine, 68*(September). Retrieved January 31, 2009, from http://www.cyc-net.org/cyc-online/cycol-0904-smith.html

Smith, M. (2006). Don't touch. *CYC OnLine, 94*(November). Retrieved January 31, 2009, from http://www.cyc-net.org/cyc-online/cycol-0611-smith.html

Stuart, C. (2008). Shaping the rules: Child and youth care boundaries in the context of relationships. Bonsai! In G. Bellefuille & F. Ricks (Eds.), *Standing on the precipice: Inquiry into the creative potential of child and youth care practice* (pp. 135–168). Edmonton, AB: McEwan Press.

Sturrock, J. (2003). *Structuralism* (2nd ed.). Oxford, UK: Blackwell Publishers.

Tompkins-Rosenblatt, P. (2004). Planning ahead: Relationships and power. *Relational Child and Youth Care Practice, 17*(2), 33–38.

Values and Ethics in Child and Youth Care Practice

SUMMARY. The implications of the practitioner's personal values are explored in relation to the professional issues of child and youth care practice. Values are inevitably a component of decision-making and therefore are integrally connected to ethics in the field. The prevalence of subjectivity over objectivity is emphasized in relation to in-the-moment decision-making for practitioners. This results in an elevated importance for the process of critical reflection with respect to personal values. The ethics of child and youth care practice are explored from both systemic and in-the-moment perspectives. The role of codes of ethics is explored as well as ethics in relation to self care and professional development, everyday preparation and practice and ethics in relation to team dynamics and functioning.

KEYWORDS. Bias, decision-making, ethics, judgment, objectivity and subjectivity, professional issues, teamwork, values

"Values," according to Scrivens (2001, p. 39), "are the underlying thread of all healthy relationships." Given the centrality of the concept of relationship within child and youth care practice, it is clear that values are an important element of that practice; so much so that it is difficult imagining child and youth care practice unfolding in the absence of any role for values. But how can we understand that role? And what is the relationship between the values we hold and the work that we do? Ultimately, why does an exploration of the professional issues of child and youth care practice require us to contemplate our values?

Part of the answer relates to the importance of Self within our practice. If we can accept the premise that Self matters, then we also have to accept the idea that so much of what we do with children, youth and families is related, in some way, to ourselves. Our value systems are informed at a minimum by the following:

• Our past—heritage, experiences, trauma and memories;
• Our present—identity questions, performance anxiety and relationship quandaries;
• Our future—fear and anxiety, expectations and hope, connections to our present and past.

In comparing our past, present and future with those of other practitioners, we quickly realize the inevitability of difference; none of us are exactly alike, and none of us hold exactly the same values. Often there are similarities in value systems or sets of values held by individuals from similar cultures or similar socioeconomic backgrounds or even similar educational backgrounds, but when examined more closely, even such similarities cannot negate the differences amongst us and our values. Given those differences, it is inevitable that in order to be engaged with children and youth we either allow our values to provide the framework for our thoughts and actions in an unfettered manner or each of us agrees to mitigate or transcend specific values in order to limit the range of acceptable interventions and interactions. If indeed we allow for the unfettered presence and impact of values in our work, the risk of exposing or impacting children and youth with harmful or negative interventions is great. For many individuals, for example, corporal punishment is deeply embedded not only as an acceptable practice but also as a core component of the value system related to raising and disciplining children. As a profession, however, child and youth care practice does not accept the value system endorsing corporal punishment. The profession of child and youth care practice has taken a stand in favor of mitigating the impact of our personal values by delineating what is acceptable and what is not, what is right and what is wrong. In so doing, the field of child and youth care practice has embraced the centrality of ethics as a guiding principle for the profession. In this sense, ethics in child and youth care serves to bridge the differences within our personal values and value systems on the one hand, and the rights and well being of children and youth as determined by a broad social, legal and cultural consensus about the rules and methods of professional engagement with children and youth on the other hand.

VALUES INFLUENCING INTERVENTIONS

There are many different kinds of rationales for promoting specific interventions with children and youth. Certainly one rationale relates to the expected outcomes of the intervention; ideally, as child and youth care practitioners, we are aware that some interventions have an evidence-base while others have been demonstrated to be ineffective. In practice, however, in-the-moment interventions have not been subject to extensive research and generally are not, in isolation at least, evidence-based. Evidence-based practices are typically more broadly articulated; practices that are compatible with cognitive-behavioral theory or that unfold within the context of human relationships can claim to have an evidence-base in the research literature. In most cases, however, in-the-moment interventions are very specific to the circumstances and can only minimally be related to a concrete evidence base. Often, it is the habitual application of in-the-moment interventions that forms the basis of rules and behavior management approaches promoted by practitioners as effective or "tried and true." In these cases, it is worthwhile to reflect on the rationale for such rules and approaches, because it often turns out that these are based on deeply embedded value systems reflecting the practitioner's past, present or even future.

There are many examples of rule discussions that turn out to be little more than differences in practitioners' value systems. A standard routine in residential programs relates to the morning wake ups of residents. A common problem associated with this routine unfolds when some residents are slow to respond to the practitioner's wake-up call. Chronic unresponsiveness and resultant lateness for breakfast and school frequently results in disagreements amongst residential practitioners how best to support the resident in changing this behavior. Some practitioners argue that at least in the case of adolescents, it is best to purchase an alarm clock and then allow the adolescent to determine his own wake up routines. The natural consequence of an ineffective wake up routine will be that he misses breakfast and potentially will be late for school. Other practitioners argue that too much is at stake for the adolescent to be left to his own devices, and that the team of practitioners instead should work harder to get this resident going in the morning, perhaps through repeated wake-up calls or with positive incentives.

There is no evidence that would specifically support either of these approaches. It is likely the case that each approach could be effective in addressing this particular problem with some adolescents but not others. And yet practitioners are typically quite adamant that their approach is the correct one. Reflecting on the rationale for maintaining one's position within this disagreement, it quickly becomes clear that this is not an issue of effective child and youth care practice but, instead, it is a discussion about values that typically reflect the practitioners' past and their own experiences as adolescents. For some, promoting early self determination and autonomy, combined with the natural consequences of making mistakes, reflects a deeply held value about individual responsibility and accountability. For others, the promotion of nurture and active assistance reflects values of protective childhoods and adult responsibility toward children and youth.

Other values could also be of relevance in this scenario. For some practitioners, the lack of cooperation during morning routines is interpreted as a form of resistance or disobedience, and some practitioners take great exception to this kind of behavior. From a different perspective, some practitioners may interpret the challenges during morning routines as a passive expression of the young person's individuality and his potential need for a different schedule that respects his need for more sleep in the mornings. What is of importance in this scenario is not so much the rationale itself, or the value system informing the rationale, but the presence of a self-reflective process that takes into account the practitioner's values and mitigates these by re-focusing a team discussion on the needs of the particular client and his particular circumstances.

In a nonresidential context, examples of value-based decision-making abound as well. As a practitioner assigned to working with a family in their home, one might encounter a situation where alcohol is offered as part of a celebration or special event for the family. For the practitioner, this poses a dilemma, as there typically would be policies from the employer that prohibit the consumption of alcohol while at work. On the other hand, participating in the celebration of the family would appear as an important step in building a relationship, and refusing the alcohol might not be helpful and place the practitioner on the outside of the family event. While a decision about whether or not to accept the offer of alcohol under these circumstances may well be rationalized around professional integrity issues or even employment issues, in reality this too represents a value-based decision for the practitioner.

Our values are often challenged by broader organizational issues and belief systems. Faith-based agencies frequently impose values on issues such as birth control, abortion and sexual orientation. Some organizations promote law and order agendas with respect to youth conduct, resulting in an expectation that practitioners seek police involvement wherever possible. Other organizations place greater value on providing youth with opportunities for learning from their mistakes and exploring alternative resolutions to criminal or quasi-criminal conduct. Child and youth care practitioners are often in positions where their own values clash with those held by the employer, resulting in dilemmas related to following the rules of the employer versus practices that are based on deeply held values and the practitioner's best estimation as to the client's needs and best interests.

In some articulations of child and youth care practice, practitioners are encouraged to allow their own values to take precedence over employer values even where the resultant practice may clash substantially with societal norms and expectations, and sometimes even the law. The Mayhem Collective, for example, openly promotes law-skirting and ethically controversial practices so long as they address the needs of youth in a very immediate context (Moen, Little, & Burnett, 2005). Others promote a "radical" approach to child and youth care practice that encourages practitioners to deconstruct the value-systems informing current practices and policies and procedures, often articulated as reflections of capitalism and historical materialism, and replacing that value system with a radical articulation of practice premised on poststructuralism and an abandonment of orthodox methods of control (Scott-Myhre, 2006).

In practice, these re-formulations of child and youth care practice and principles result in greater interest in restorative justice approaches, harm reduction strategies and advocacy on behalf of self determination and a re-claiming of identities. From the perspective of the practitioner, however, all of these challenges to current practices and employer or broader system expectations are reflections of competing value systems, and it is not always easy for the practitioner to find his way around this complex web of value statements, value judgments and value-based decisions. And yet, "value confusion" is no reason to be overly concerned. What really matters is not so much any specific value system but one's awareness of that value system and its impact on decision-making and interventions. It is in this context that the practitioner encounters the "problem of objectivity" in child and youth care practice, and this is what we will explore next.

OBJECTIVITY AND SUBJECTIVITY IN CHILD AND YOUTH CARE PRACTICE

No matter what our past and present may be about, it is not inherently problematic that there is something profoundly personal about the work we do; it becomes problematic only when we ignore this and pretend that we have the ability to work with children, youth and families in an "objective" manner. There are two reasons why objectivity is simply not possible in child and youth are practice:

1. We are human beings with specific values and perspectives that are derived at least in part from our past and present, and no two child and youth care practitioners have identical values and perspectives; and
2. Given that our work unfolds primarily through the medium of relationship, child and youth care practitioners are *organic* components of the work itself. Objectivity implies standing on the outside and looking in, but since we are already on the inside, we cannot simultaneously move outside.

It is extremely important to distinguish objectivity and subjectivity within our practice. Without such distinction, many of the core assumptions within our profession become vulnerable. For example, we have long ago agreed that child and youth care practitioners are unique individuals and that it is extremely important for each practitioner to explore their Self. If indeed we were able to perform our duties in an entirely objective manner, there would really be no point to exploring one's Self; the work would be disconnected from our own existence. Similarly, within the context of relationships, we are aware not only of the give and take characterizing all relationships but also of the spaces "in-between" the practitioner and the child or youth (Garfat, 2008), and we recognize that these spaces are shaped by the individuality and identity of the practitioner and the child, on the one hand, and the mutual responses between these individualities and identities, on the other hand. If indeed we were able to be objective, there would not be any reason to consider that mutual interaction between identities, since the practitioner's identity would be outside of the relationship.

Subjectivity, on the other hand, allows us to incorporate our values, biases and judgment into the relationships we have with children and youth, and by doing so we can mitigate their potentially harmful effects. In reality, we cannot simply abandon our belief systems during the time we are at work, especially given the constant mutuality of interactions with children and youth. Abandoning our belief systems and our values would leave us profoundly vulnerable to being "overtaken" by corporate or unbalanced value systems designed to impose control and establish truth—predetermined ways of being, of conducting oneself and of managing change and growth.

There are many examples in child and youth care practice contexts that relate to the distinctions between objectivity and subjectivity. In residential care, point and level systems are reflective of the belief that there can indeed be an objective approach to working with children and youth. These systems assume that every child will respond in particular ways to rewards and consequences and to gaining privileges and suffering losses. In this framing of child and youth care practice, the practitioner is removed entirely from the change process of the child or youth and really takes on the role of accountant or operator with respect to the child (Pazaratz, 2009). In family work, approaches that stress the importance of holding families responsible for following through on goals and expectations at the exclusion of work stressing experiential and relational approaches to "being" with families are reflective of a belief in objectivity as well. Much like point and level systems, the practitioner's role is reduced to being in charge of evaluating and judging the performance of the family. In educational settings, "objective" approaches match children and youth with learning tools that are deemed effective in addressing specific learning needs. Again, the individuality of the child or youth is side-lined in favor of an objective assessment of the problem and the imposition of a solution that "ought to work." The assignment of a child and youth care practitioner to a young person with behavioral challenges is deemed an "objective" response; the young person's thoughts on who he would like to be with is largely irrelevant.

Subjectivity allows us to recognize that our presence, regardless of the tools we use in our work, is itself impacted by our biases and our judgments. Rather than pretending that we can rise above these, recognizing our subjectivity in practice allows us to expose our biases and judgments to responses from the child or youth and to make adjustments to how we manage these as we continue to be present and engaged with the child. While we may not like acknowledging that we have biases or that we engage in judgment, each of these concepts becomes much more benign if we are able to work with them openly and honestly.

Biases

Everybody holds biases, but most of the time, such biases are not articulated or acknowledged. Biases are deeply held preferences that are based on an assumptive truth. One of the reasons we often do not acknowledge our biases, even to ourselves, is that they are not based on facts or evidence; if we were challenged on our biases, we would not likely be able to defend them in a particularly compelling manner. At a very general level, biases can determine our preferences in terms of what kinds of clients we like to work with, what kinds of personalities we might be drawn to, and how we might manage loyalty conflicts. Many child and youth care practitioners, for example, can readily identify specific client profiles that are of interest and others that are not of interest. Often, practitioners have a bias against working with sexual offenders, perhaps because the practitioner has not yet resolved the inherent tension between the damage done to others by the offender, on the one hand, and his need for assistance or treatment, and potentially his earlier victimization, on the other hand. Other practitioners may hold a bias against children or youth expressing their pain through difficult behaviors. In this case, they may not be able to distinguish between a child or youth's personality and their way of communicating pain, discomfort or a lack of well-being. And again, other practitioners may simply not be able to resolve the tension between remaining supportive to colleagues, on the one hand, and supporting children or youth through conflict with colleagues, on the other hand.

There are an infinite number of possibilities with respect to biases, and these do creep into virtually every aspect of the practitioner's work. Our preferences with respect to clients, work contexts or managing human relationships are deeply embedded, and such preferences speak to who we are as individuals and how we resolve our own experiences and identity factors in relation to the issues and challenges presenting themselves in the work we do. Simple biases are not inherently problematic so long as we are able to remain conscious of having such biases and willing to reflect on their impact. It is when we fail to do this and instead allow our biases to be expressed as judgment that we create problems within our practice that have greater implications for the well-being of our clients.

Judgment

Not all biases result in judgment, but judgment is always the outcome of bias. Once we are engaged in judgment, we have allowed whatever biases we may hold to take on an expressive character, one that determines not only our feelings toward a particular person or issue but also whether that person or issue is right or wrong, legitimate or not, acceptable or unacceptable. Judgment is the result of a seemingly irreconcilable difference between the values we hold and our perception of other people's values, identities or behaviors.

Some judgments are obviously malignant and reflect broader themes of racism, sexism, homophobia and other identity-based rejections of others. These judgments are difficult to overcome because they are almost always very deeply entrenched in the individual's conscience and reinforced by that individual's interpretation of social dynamics and messages. For example, a practitioner's judgment of Black youth as criminals or untrustworthy become reinforced by the often unbalanced reporting of crime statistics or specific criminal events involving black youth. Unlike biases, it is much more difficult to find safe spaces to explore one's racism with the support of colleagues or supervisors because racism is deemed unacceptable and often excluded as a topic of exploration amongst professionals. The net result is that the judgment associated with the practitioner's racism is never really challenged or confronted, nor is the practitioner afforded the opportunity to explore the roots of that racism.

Most judgment, however, is much less obvious than racism or other identity-based judgments and reflects a much more nuanced movement from bias to judgment. Behavioral patterns, lack of follow through on commitments, an apparent lack of motivation and irresponsible decision-making all are examples of situations or themes that may fall prey to our judgment. It is one thing to redirect poor behavior or use strategies to promote better choices; but it is quite another thing to judge a young person for failing to comply or for failing to perform. Once such judgment takes hold, practitioners will be less able to maintain their focus on being present with the young person because the young person is now someone to be rejected and, perhaps, corrected. Judgment in child and youth care practice reflects the failure to remain transparent about one's biases, and the impact of such judgment can be quite destructive. All of the core principles of child and youth care practice, such as relationships, caring and engagement become vulnerable and threatened in the presence of judgment because these principles rely substantially on the practitioner's capacity and desire to be present with the young person through a mutual process of discovery and identity-formation both for the practitioner and the young person.

FROM VALUES TO ETHICS

The relationship between values and ethics in child and youth care practice is a complex one. While the field of ethics is, without a doubt, based on an articulation of broad social values, it is not simply an adaptation of such values for the purpose of guiding practice. Ethics in our profession frame our responsibilities toward children, youth and their families based on what is right and wrong in the specific context of intervening in their lives. Intervention in this context does not only refer to specific activities or identifiable actions but also to our passive presence and to the manifestations of our relationships with children, youth and their families. It is therefore necessary to consider the ethics of our practice on many different dimensions, including:

• Protecting the rights of children and youth;
• Acting with knowledge and understanding of good practice;

- Prioritizing the well-being of children and youth over our loyalties to colleagues and other adults;
- Empowering children, youth and families with respect to self determination, identity formation, privacy and personal autonomy.

There are many circumstances where ethical practice becomes compromised by competing value systems, and such compromises are articulated through rationalizations that typically reflect the practitioner's personal value system. Withholding information about pregnancy termination choices, for example, or about practices or themes reflecting a young person's cultural or religious heritage, are symptomatic of practitioners rationalizing unethical practices within the context of their own value systems. In order to mitigate the potential for such unethical practices, professional ethics in child and youth care practice, as well as other disciplines such as social work, nursing and early childhood education, reflect themes and guidelines that transcend the client-centered dimensions of ethical conduct cited above and include also systemic, sectoral and organizational dimensions of ethical conduct.

ETHICS IN CHILD AND YOUTH CARE PRACTICE

The subject of ethics manifests itself within our discipline in myriad ways (Greenwald, 2007; Modlin, 2006; Ricks, 1997; Ricks & Garfat, 1998). Wherever the discipline is organized by means of an association, child and youth care practitioners are subject to a Code of Ethics. Practitioners also encounter ethics with respect to systemic issues pursuant to the institutions providing services to children and youth. And they encounter ethics in their day-to-day decision-making. In fact, while ethics may not be a daily conversation topic in our field, in reality it is the foundation of everything we do. This is the premise of Garfat and Ricks's (1995) argument that ethics in our field are "self-driven." This is also reflected in the conversational representations of ethical reflection presented by Greenwald (2007, 2008). There is an expressed hope within our field that our actions are driven by considerations of ethics and that practitioners are aware and conscious of the role of ethics in their day-to-day work.

Codes of Ethics

In most places where there are child and youth care practitioners, there is also an association seeking to regulate and promote the discipline. In Canada, 9 out of 10 provinces have their own provincial association, and each of these has developed a Code of Ethics. There is also a national umbrella organization called the *Council of Canadian Child and Youth Care Associations*, which provides a coordinating function for all of the provincial associations. In the United States, there are several state-based associations as well, some with their own code of ethics and some without. Currently, the momentum for organizational infrastructure in the United States rests with the *North American Certification Project*, which seeks to develop and maintain standards of knowledge and practice amongst practitioners in both Canada and the United States (Mattingly, 2002). Child and Youth Care associations also are in place in other parts of the world, most notably South Africa, Israel, the United Kingdom and Australia. Each has its own Code of Ethics, some of which are quite long and extensive while others are short and cover only some basic principles.

An immediate problem with the Codes of Ethics in all child and youth care jurisdictions is the lack of enforcement that pertains to these. In fact, there is not a single jurisdiction anywhere in the world where child and youth workers are required to be members of an association and to abide by the Code of Ethics developed by that association (although there are some employers who do have this requirement). In practice, child and youth care practitioners are subject to an employer's code of conduct and where it exists, perhaps an employer's own code of ethics. In the latter scenario, the employer's code of ethics most commonly is derived from the principles contained in the Codes of Ethics of other, generally more recognized, social work.

A Code of Ethics typically spells out, in writing, the core principles of ethical practice, and as such, it makes reference to the nature of conduct, the type of knowledge, and the relationship with other professionals that ought to be followed by practitioners. In this sense, Codes of Ethics in our discipline are not much different than those in related disciplines such as social work. A major difference between child and youth care and other disciplines, however, is the degree of recognition awarded to the practitioners by institutions and employers.

Given that this continues to be lacking in our discipline, the onus for abiding by the Code of Ethics rests primarily with the practitioner herself. This can be highly problematic, since several of the core principles enshrined in the Code of Ethics in child and youth care are resource intensive and therefore are difficult to abide by without employer support.

By way of example, we can consider the principle of best practice based on current knowledge and research which most Codes of Ethics require the practitioner to maintain by means of ongoing professional development activities. While most practitioners would undoubtedly be happy to oblige, the reality is that this requires a professional development program sponsored by the employer that is sufficiently extensive to support keeping up with a rapidly evolving and developing discipline. Yet there is very little evidence to suggest that employers of child and youth care practitioners support this level of professional development. Field specific conferences regularly suffer from poor attendance on the part of front-line practitioners (as a result of costs, not motivation), few employers make available research material or professional journals covering the discipline, and training and professional development events that are supported by the employer primarily unfold within the parameters of different disciplines.

The Code of Ethics of the *Ontario Association of Child and Youth Counsellors* stipulates that "we will only enter into contracts that allow us to maintain our professional integrity" (Ontario Association of Child and Youth Counsellors, 1985); again, we can readily identify the reliance on the employer in terms of upholding this principle. While we might be able to make choices about our conduct and approaches to specific service situations, as employees we are not likely to have too much choice about the contracts we enter. Moreover, this particular principle may, on occasion, clash with another principle of the Code: "We will develop, implement, and administer the policies and procedures of our respective agencies and institutions"; to the extent that the contracts we enter into in our work are indeed determined by the employer, it may become difficult to decline such contracts when we feel our professional integrity is threatened while also abiding by the need to implement the policies and procedures of our employer.

In practice, a Code of Ethics provides very little direction for the practitioner in terms of every day decision-making. Codes specific to the discipline of child and youth care practice are often unknown by the employer and very rarely make it onto the agenda of team or supervisory discussions. The generality of such Codes also does not provide enough concrete information or guidance for the practitioner to remain conscious of ethical considerations in practice settings. For this reason, much of the discussion about ethics in child and youth care practice is premised less on the written and formal articulations of Codes of Ethics and more on contemplations about virtue and open-ended values for the practitioner (Austin & Halpin, 2007; Kidder, 2005; Peterson & Seligman, 2004).

Ethical Issues at the Systemic Level

Child and youth care practitioners work in environments where decisions are made every day based on myriad considerations and not always with ethics at the forefront of decision-making. The reality is that child and youth care typically unfolds within an institutional context that is resource dependent and that is subject to all of the dynamics associated with institutional identity and ambition. As a result, many of the scenarios faced by child and youth care practitioners are themselves the result of decisions that lack in ethical quality. In this context, considerations of ethics encounter their nemesis—considerations of bureaucratic needs and bureaucratic process.

The core of all institutional strategies is self preservation. The bureaucracy developed by institutions serves the purpose of ensuring self preservation through the development of policies and procedures that manage the precarious balance of resources, service goals and risk. It follows, therefore, that the fundamental component of ethical conduct for child and youth workers, typically articulated as the centrality of the client and her well being, is always at risk of being overshadowed by considerations of institutional goals and needs. The nature of relationships, the degree of investment, admission and discharge decisions, as well as the level of comfort provided in physical care environments all are a function of decision-making at the institutional level. This does not mean that the child and youth care practitioner has no role at all in these matters, but it does mean that the possibilities are considerably limited by institutional dynamics over which the practitioner typically has minimal control.

It is possible to divide the ethical issues at the systemic level into those where the practitioner has virtually no control versus those where the practitioner does have some control and where decision-making can resolve ethical dilemmas at least to the degree that it can remove the practitioner from questionable ethics (but not always to the degree that such ethical dilemmas are resolved in favor of the client). The former type of ethical issues might include:

Hiring of Staff—the hiring of unqualified or poorly suited personnel;
Termination of Staff—disciplinary processes and human resource decisions;
Physical Infrastructure—the degree of investment and even the choice of location of service sites;
Hours of Operation—when service can be delivered, employment laws or union rules related to scheduling;
Admission Decisions—assessment of referrals and matching of clients;
Wait Lists—management of waitlists and decisions about prioritizing within the wait lists;
Risk Management—discharge decisions based on client conduct, as well as policies related to liability issues, such as touching of clients, boundaries generally;
Capacity—decisions about enrolment and over-enrolment.

This list could undoubtedly be expanded to cover scenarios and decisions specific to particular sectors and life spaces of children and youth. The essential point in considering the items on this list is the degree to which decision-making at the institutional level can impact the ethical scenarios facing the child and youth care practitioner. It is of course true that any practitioner could simply walk away from institutions that make decisions based on bureaucratic needs in order to avoid ethical dilemmas in her own work; the challenge is that in virtually all institutional contexts these ethical dilemmas appear, leaving as the only option for the practitioner a career change. In spite of this rather bleak outlook with respect to ethics in our field, there are many scenarios where the practitioner does have some choices, and these too are worthy of consideration (Elsdon, 1998; Garfat & Ricks, 1995; White, 2004):

Rules Based on Culture or Religion

In many service settings, practitioners encounter ethical dilemmas that are specifically related to the cultural or faith-based policy context of the employer. Catholic organizations, for example, frequently have policies about sexual orientation, pregnancy prevention, and abortion that might not coincide with the practitioner's outlook. In these circumstances, avoiding employment in such organizations is indeed a choice the practitioner can make. One might argue that seeking employment in such organizations while aware of the potential ethical dilemmas that are likely to arise, is in and of itself an unethical decision on the part of the practitioner.

Rules Based on Risk Management Strategies

Where the practitioner encounters risk management strategies that prohibit practices considered vital for the healthy growth of children, such as no touch policies, again the choice of leaving the employer is present, and again the practitioner must act in accordance with her ethical standards in deciding whether this kind of work environment is the right choice. Given that there are organizations that do not manage risk in this manner, it is reasonable to place the onus on the practitioner to make an ethical decision.

Self-care and Professional Development

Both of these feature prominently within the Codes of Ethics developed by associations and professional groups. As discussed earlier, the onus cannot be entirely on the practitioner in abiding by these ethical requirements, but this does not absolve the practitioner from her responsibilities in this respect either. In reality, practitioners can choose to seek out employment opportunities where self care and professional development enjoy greater support from the employer, and they can, at least in some measure, pursue self care and professional development activities independently through cost free or minimal cost resources that are publicly available in libraries or on line. Failure to take any action when faced with a lack of support in these areas becomes an issue of ethics precisely because the practitioner does have some choices and capacities to act.

Ethics at the systemic level are difficult to manage for the practitioner, but this does not mean that such ethics can be ignored. As a field of practice, we are faced with imperfect scenarios, but we also have opportunities to act in ways that correspond to our ethical standards and that may even send a clear message to employers and institutions that our field is not one to conform to norms and procedures that fail to place the client at the center of our activities. Beyond these ethical issues at the systems level, child and youth care practitioners encounter ethical issues at the front line level as well, and it is to these that we now turn our attention.

ETHICAL ISSUES EVERY DAY

It is important to make a distinction between decisions that reflect poor practice or limited competence versus those that reflect an inadequate consideration of ethics. Any decision can be evaluated in terms of "right" or "wrong," but that does not mean that all decisions we make as practitioners are decisions about ethics. It may not be "right" to impose an early bedtime on a child because she has difficulty settling at night, but it is not inherently unethical; although it might be unethical if we are motivated to impose this consequence for reasons that reflect our needs more so than those of the child. It may also not be "right" to plan activities that regularly exclude some children or youth as a result of lack of interest or perceived lack of skills, but it is not unethical to do so, unless we are excluding these children or youth for reasons that reflect our needs and preferences.

Ethics are about intention and motivation more so than about effectiveness or outcomes, although if outcomes are poor over a sustained period of time, one might consider there to be an ethical responsibility to change one's approach. Certainly within a utilitarian perspective of ethics, outcomes do serve an important function in judging ethical merit. In the day to day work of child and youth care practitioners, ethics are also about the efforts we make in providing the services we claim to offer to children and youth. As such, ethical issues appear every day, and even moment to moment, in child and youth care practice, and often child and youth care practitioners are quite oblivious to the ethical consequences of their decisions and actions. In order to bring these issues to life, we will explore every day ethics in several practice contexts. First, we will explore ethics related to how we prepare ourselves for what we do. Second, we will look at ethics as they relate to team dynamics. And finally, we will examine the ethical foundation of relationships.

Everyday Preparation

Child and youth care practitioners are not perfect, and it ought to be understood that everyday activities and decisions will not "cure" the child or the youth. It ought to also be clear that child and youth care practitioners will every day do things and make decisions that in hindsight will be understood as "wrong," "ill-conceived," or simply ineffective. Making mistakes is part of the job. On the other hand, child and youth care practitioners do know what the purpose of their presence is, why they are in the job, what their actions and decisions hope to achieve, and what the fundamental goals of the program are. And child and youth care practitioners do know that they are required to promote the well being of the child and take actions and make decisions that are consistent with this mandate. Regardless of the specific approach to the work promoted by the employer, and regardless of the policies and procedures that must be followed, all settings where child and youth care practitioners are employed aim to assist children and youth in some way, and all such settings hope to avoid harming children and youth.

The failure to prepare oneself adequately to ensure that there is at least a possibility of assisting children and that the possibility of harming children is minimized is indeed an ethical issue. Obvious examples of unethical preparation include appearing at the work site under the influence of drugs or alcohol. Doing so significantly reduces the chances of assisting children and also significantly increases the chances of harming children. It is therefore not only irresponsible to do so, but it is also unethical.

There are many less obvious steps in preparing oneself to be present with children and youth. Ensuring enough sleep prior to the shift, considering what to wear given planned activities, being conscious of special circumstances for particular children (such as birthdays, graduations, anniversaries of major losses) and preparing ways to acknowledge these prior to arrival at work are all examples that undoubtedly reflect good practice but also reflect ethical conduct.

The standard by which an issue shifts from a quality of practice issue to an ethical issue is determined by what we know and what we therefore ought to be prepared for. It is knowingly failing to prepare oneself to maximize the opportunities to be helpful to children and youth that create an opening for ethical vulnerability. And likewise, it is knowingly failing to prepare ourselves in such a way that we minimize the possibility of harm to children and youth that shifts poor practice to unethical conduct.

Everyday Ethics of Teams

Child and youth care practice often unfolds in the context of team work; this is certainly the case in residential settings, but it is also true in many other kinds of settings, such as special education classrooms, hospitals, community centers, drop-in programs, after-school programs and mainstream schools. Working on a team presents special opportunities and special challenges for individual practitioners. An obvious opportunity relates to the resources presented by team approaches: more varied skills and knowledge, potentially greater cultural competence, multiple personalities, someone to listen and someone to vent to and de-brief with, and a system of accountability that provides for much greater vigilance than individual supervisors. For every opportunity, however, there are challenges. Teams should serve to provide accountability for individual practitioners, but they can also serve the purpose of diminishing accountability. Loyalty to teams and to particular team members can conflict with loyalty to children and youth.

The presence of teams introduces adult dynamics into child or youth-serving environments. This is a significant observation, because adult dynamics are not typically any more or any less functional and positive than dynamics amongst children and youth or between children and youth and specific adults. Inter-personal conflict, issues of intimacy and boundaries, professional disagreements, perceptions of incompetence, personal likes and dislikes, judgment, racism, sexism, homophobia, competition and a host of other issues and problems emerge when adults try to work together toward a common goal.

Effective teamwork requires a great deal of effort on the part of every team member, and it also requires open and honest communication, a strong sense of and a shared vision of professional conduct, and, more than anything else, a common vision for ethical conduct. In practice, not nearly enough time is spent ensuring that this hard work is actually done, jointly as a team and individually by every practitioner. Supervisors do what they can to provide leadership in this process, but they are not around when teams work together, think together and make decisions together. As a result, everyday ethics of teams become vulnerable to some of the weaknesses of adult collaboration.

One of the core ethical issues in this respect relates to the concept of loyalty. Who should the practitioner be loyal to in times of conflict between worker and child? Does advocacy for the child trump support for the team? Can a colleague be disempowered in order to empower a child? Can we intervene when we witness a colleague engaging with a child inappropriately? Can we overturn the decisions of the team if we feel differently about the circumstances that led to the decision in the first place? These are only some of the endless questions that can be raised with respect to the loyalty dilemma in practice environments. Ultimately, the ethical issue contained in team dynamics is the degree to which the interests of the child take precedence over the interests of the team. One complicating factor is that in many cases, it *is* in the interest of the child to maintain the interests of the team, even if in the moment the child appears unhappy or disadvantaged. Where to draw the line?

Once again, the everyday ethics of teams are reflective of the motivations and intentions of our decisions. Supporting a colleague at the expense of a client *may* be ethical, but only if such support is motivated by an honest (although not necessarily accurate) evaluation of the interests of the child. It may indeed be ethical to allow a colleague to complete an inappropriate engagement with a child and confront the colleague about this later, but if one perceived such engagement to be harmful to the child, it becomes unethical to do so and we are ethically bound to intervene in the moment. The point is that everyday ethics of teams are determined by the moment-to-moment circumstances that arise, not by any pre-set assumptions about the need to maintain the integrity of the team. Teams are a support structure for the delivery of services, not a space of entitlement. Ethics require us to focus on the services and their connections to the clients, not on the support structures in place to deliver these services.

One aspect of teams that rarely is mentioned in the context of ethics is the very deeply entrenched belief that teams must maintain consistency at all costs. In fact, a great deal of team discord is the result of accusations amongst team members that the command of consistency has been breached. This leads to very important barriers to ethical conduct. Consistency may well be beneficial for children and youth who have experienced primarily chaos and instability in their lives. And so long as consistency is seen as promoting such benefits for children and youth, there are no ethical concerns. It is when consistency becomes an end in itself, something to be maintained because the team demands it, that we build a foundation for unethical behavior. This is the foundation for denying children their individuality, for imposing on children rules and expectations that are not geared to their strengths or their interests, and for abandoning any meaningful attempt to build up the resilience of the children and youth we serve. Consistency is only one of many concepts that can, under some circumstances, have benefits. But promoting consistency *on behalf of the team* is reflective of a decisive victory of the team over the children in the loyalty dilemma discussed earlier.

Everyday Ethics of Relationships

Child and youth care practice unfolds through the medium of relationship. Relationships have characteristics and attributes that provide the foundation for all kinds of ethical dilemmas. Perhaps the most obvious example of such dilemmas relates to the concept of boundaries. While there are many variations in how we constitute our boundaries with respect to specific clients, it is fair to assume that virtually all child and youth care practitioners consider the professional implications of their boundaries. In this sense, our relationships at work are not entirely the same as our private or our intimate relationships. Love, friendship, and other kinds of personal bonds are firmly within the realm of the private; our relationships with the kids we work with are characterized more by treatment goals, the desire to build resilience, and the hope of making the experience of children or youth receiving service as positive as possible. Therefore, whatever limitations we create are typically created for the sake of advancing the interests of the child or youth.

The ethical dilemmas emerge when it is not entirely clear what those interests of the child or youth might be. In the classic scenario often used in classrooms, a youth who has experienced something traumatic asks the child and youth care worker for a cigarette. In thinking about the scenario, questions emerge whether giving the cigarette to the youth is the right thing or the wrong thing to do. Some might argue that withholding the cigarette might prevent an important opportunity to explore the trauma the youth has experienced. Others point to the fact that providing a cigarette to a person under the age of 19 (in Ontario) is illegal, and surely we would not want to endorse illegal activity in front of a youth.

There are virtually unlimited scenarios that unfold in the day to day work of child and youth workers where ethical dilemmas manifest themselves. A child and youth care practitioner working with families in their homes might be offered a glass of wine while being in the home. The policies of her employer prohibit the consumption of alcohol while at work. Taking the wine might be a good way of connecting with the family, but it would constitute a breach of policy; not taking the wine might be taken as a rejection of the family's customs, and this might render the work less effective. So what is the right thing to do?

These kinds of ethical dilemmas are difficult to resolve. In most cases, there probably is no right answer that would fit every conceivable situation. In fact, one way of resolving these dilemmas is to embrace the idea that every client (child or family) is unique, and that the role of a child and youth care practitioner is to embrace that uniqueness and join the client wherever no immediate harm can be identified. Doing so, however, still poses some difficult ethical issues, particularly because making decisions about breaching employer policies and procedures violates one of the principles enshrined within most Codes of Ethics in the profession ("we will abide by the policies and procedures of the employer").

The everyday ethics of relationships are not limited, however, to what we *do* within the context of our relationships. The very concept of relationship presents some ethical dilemmas and obligations inasmuch as it implies commitment. We know that when we engage clients in relationships, we will eventually have to terminate these relationships as the client is discharged from the service. Our relationships are specific to our employment context and the client's involvement within that context. This mitigates the kind of commitment we are able to make to the client when we first start offering ourselves within the context of relationships. Given the significant impact of loss of relationship, how do we ethically justify our offering of a relationship we know we will have to terminate? Are we setting the client up for loss? Perhaps the answer to this dilemma lies in how we use the concept of relationship in our work with clients and also how we articulate this to the client. We might have a reasonable understanding of what relationship means in our professional context, but we certainly cannot assume that the client will share that understanding. The need for us to be clear, therefore, about the nature of relationship we are offering becomes an ethical responsibility. Without such clarity, our relationship-based approach to the work becomes just another disguise for deception and dishonesty.

One way around all of this is to abandon the language of relationship altogether and instead adopt the language of relational work. This is a relatively new development in the field, and although it did not evolve from ethical considerations, it provides an opportunity to resolve at least one part of the everyday ethics related to relationships. Relational work differs from relationship-based work in two major ways: first, it does not assume the presence of a "relationship condition"; in other words, we do not *have* relationships, but we engage our clients *relationally*. This means that rather than offering a way of being related to one another, we are engaging the client in being together when we are both present. Second, the target for commitment in relationship-based work is the relationship itself, which, as we discussed, is difficult to sustain. In relational work, in contrast, the target of commitment is the space between ourselves and the client whenever we are present together. This type of commitment is very intense, but it reflect the emphasis of "in the moment" so characteristic of our discipline, rather than the imposed presumptive framework of relationship (Garfat, 2008).

CRITICAL REFLECTION AND ETHICS

Ethics in all professions that are about human interactions and relationships are complex and rarely offer clarity or obvious ways to proceed. In child and youth care practice, ethical issues are present both within the structural contexts of our workplaces and within the everyday experiences with colleagues and clients. It is generally much easier to deconstruct the ethics of someone else's actions than it is to set an ethical standard of practice for oneself. This is why critical reflection is one of the most important responsibilities of practitioners. All the theory notwithstanding, once we are engaged with a client or a group of clients, our activities and interventions accelerate, and our time to think is sharply reduced. Practicalities and operational considerations often take over and keeping one's head above water just to keep up can be challenging. Yet, if we fail to reflect critically on the work we have done, on our relationships with clients, on the trouble spots we encountered throughout the day and on the collaboration we experienced with our colleagues, we are very likely going to allow our subjectivities to go unchecked, with no real understanding of the impact.

Critical reflection is our most valuable tool in mitigating the myriad contexts in which values and ethics collide in our moment to moment practice. It is really the only way in which can learn from the varied and often unpredictable situations and scenarios we encounter in our work; it is an effective way of ensuring that we remain conscious of our subjectivities and that we find ways of integrating these into a framework of ethical conduct suitable for our specific employment context.

REFERENCES

Austin, D., & Halpin, W. (2007). The caring response. *Relational Child and Youth Care Practice, 20*(2), 62–64.

Elsdon, I. (1998). Educating toward awareness: Self-awareness in ethical decision making for child and youth care workers. *Journal of Child and Youth Care, 1*(3), 55–67.

Garfat, T. (2008). The inter-personal in-between: An exploration of relational child and youth care practice. In G. Bellefeuille & F. Ricks (Eds.), *Standing on the precipice: Inquiry into the creative potential of child and youth care practice* (pp. 7–34). Edmonton, Canada: McEwan Press.

Garfat, T., & Ricks, F. (1995). Self-driven ethical decision-making: A model for child and youth care. *Child and Youth Care Forum, 24*(6), 393–404.

Greenwald, M. (2007). Ethics is hot . . . So what? *Relational Child and Youth Care Practice, 20*(1), 27–33.

Greenwald, M. (2008). The virtuous child and youth care practitioner. In G. Bellefeuille & F. Ricks (Eds.), *Standing on the precipice: Inquiry into the creative potential of child and youth care practice* (pp. 169–204). Edmonton, Canada: McEwan Press.

Kidder, R. M. (2005). *Moral courage.* New York: Harper.

Mattingly, M. A. (2002). The North American Certification Project: Competencies for professional child and youth care practitioners. *Journal of Child and Youth Care Work, 17*, 16–49.

Modlin, H. (2006). Standards, ethics, and professional child and youth care associations. *Relational Child and Youth Care Practice, 19*(2), 54–56.

Moen, J., Little, N., & Burnett, M. (2005). The earth is dying: A radical child and youth care perspective. *Relational Child and Youth Care Practice, 18*(1), 7–13.

Ontario Association of Child and Youth Counsellors. (1985). *Code of Ethics.* Retrieved June 12, 2009, from www.oacyc.org/page4.html

Pazaratz, D. (2009). *Residential treatment of adolescents: Integrative principles and practices.* New York: Routledge.

Peterson, C., & Seligman, M. P. (2004). *Character strengths and virtues: A handbook classification.* New York: Oxford University Press.

Ricks, F. (1997). Perspectives on ethics in child and youth care. *Child and Youth Care Forum*, *26*(3), 187–204.

Ricks, F., & Garfat, T. (1998). Ethics education in child and youth care: A Canadian study. *Journal of Child and Youth Care*, *11*(4), 69–76.

Scott-Myhre, H. (2006). Radical youth work: Becoming visible. *Child and Youth Care Forum*, *35*(3), 219–229.

Scrivens, V. (2000). Values. *Journal of Child and Youth Care*, *14*(3), 39–48.

White, J. (2004). Earning their trust and keeping them safe: Exploring ethical tensions in the practice of youth suicide prevention. *Relational Child and Youth Care Practice*, *17*(3), 13–21.

Relationships with Children
and Families

SUMMARY. This article explores the professional issues of relationships within child and youth care practice. The concept of "relationship-based practice" is examined from conceptual, linguistic and power-based perspectives. It is argued that the power base of relationships amongst practitioners manifests itself along five specific contexts: institutional dynamics, culture, conventions, social expectations, and language. Relationship-based practice is compared with relational practice. It is argued that a more complex view of relationships within child and youth care practice will serve to prevent misuses and poorly defined practices on the part of practitioners. To this end, it is recommended that greater emphasis be placed within the discipline on the relational content of training and professional development activities.

KEYWORDS. Culture, institutional dynamics, power and relationships, relational practice, relationships, residential care, teamwork

Child and youth care is a discipline that unfolds through the medium of relationships. Notwithstanding the simplicity of this statement, there has been a great deal of theoretical and more practice-oriented work within our field to develop the concept of relationship in some detail and to ascertain exactly what "working through the medium of relationship" might mean. It is probably fair to say that while there is near-consensus within the literature that relationships are important and represent a core concept in child and youth care practice, it is also apparent within that literature that there are significant differences in how the concept is articulated (Austin & Halpin, 1987; Burns, 1987; Fewster, 2001a; 2001b; Maier, 1992; Parry, 1999; Shealy, 1999). More recently, there is even some questioning whether the concept of relationship accurately depicts what child and youth care practitioners do or ought to do (Garfat, 2008; Gharabaghi, 2008).

The concept of relationship was introduced to child and youth care theory and practice early in the development of the field, even well before the field became known as child and youth care. Thus, we find references to this concept in the work of Addams (1910) and Korczack (1925). It was, however, the work of some of the foundational writers of the discipline proper that advanced the position of relationship to a central one (Bettleheim, 1974; Redl, 1959; Trieschman, Whittaker, & Brendtro, 1969). By the 1970s and into the 1980s, virtually all contributions to the field included not only some reference to relationships, but much more in-depth contemplation of it and, in many cases, active promotion of a "relationship-based approach" to child and youth care (Maier, 1987). According to Krueger (1990, p. 6), "caring relationships— relationships that include empathy, trust, security, compassion and sympathy—are the foundation on which treatment is built." Brendtro, Ness and Mitchell (2005, p. 48) exclaim that "it is the strength of human bonds...not the severity of punishment that preserves human order."

The analysis of relationship took a new turn in the 1990s, when the concept of "having relationships" was challenged by the concept of "being in relationships" (Fewster, 1991). This new way of conceptualizing relationships within the practice of child and youth care corresponded to the more intense contemplation of the Self. Putting the Self at the centre of the reflective process required a re-conceptualization of relationships as a state of being rather than as a tool to be used or sidelined as the practitioner saw fit. Within this perspective, relationships were articulated as inevitable products of being with a child in his life space. Myriad other concepts also flowed from this new perspective: being present, engagement, self care, and a much more complex articulation of the concept of boundaries (Krueger, 2004, 2007; Krueger & Powell, 1990).

While there has indeed been a great deal of movement in the way in which we have contemplated the concept of relationship over the past fifty years in particular, it is important to note that much of these contemplations came out of a very specific context of the field of child and youth care: the residential context. This reflects, to a great extent, the degree to which the field itself had been largely limited to residential work for much of its history, but it also reflects the fact that most of the contributors to the field until recently were themselves employed in residential programs for children and youth early in their careers and frequently carried their employment experiences into their research agendas. Not surprisingly, therefore, we can identify today a significant trend toward associating relationship-based work with residential programs where it is perhaps most obvious that worker and child "are being" together in the life space (however temporary) of the child.

Throughout the past twenty years, however, child and youth care practitioners have been steadily increasing the breadth and scope of their employment experiences. While residential care continues to be an important employer of child and youth care practitioners, today we find these practitioners active in a host of other programs and sectors. These might include education—mainstream and special education—health care, recreation programs, community centres, specialized treatment groups such as anger management or self-esteem building groups, outreach programs and in-home family intervention or support programs. In fact, several nonresidential programs and service approaches were developed specifically as responses to what was seen as ineffective service within the residential sector. Multi-systemic Therapy (MST), family support programs (FSP), and Intensive Family Preservation Programs (IFP) all came out of a frustration with the outcomes of residential treatment services and perhaps also with shifting ideological perspectives related primarily to the enormous public funding required for such programs.

With these new developments in service delivery approaches, the field of child and youth care has had to adjust in terms of articulating relationship-based work in such a way that it could transcend the real or imagined assumptions of milieu therapy. And indeed, we find today a rapidly growing body of literature that provides analyses of relationship-based approaches in the context of education (Beck & Malley, 2003), family work (Garfat, 2003), and outreach programs (Griffin, 2008). Within this literature, the concept of relationship is slowly being replaced with the concept of "relational practice" (Garfat, 2008).

There are many specific differences between relationship-based work and relational practice, but perhaps the difference that most concerns us here is the way in which these concepts make assumptions about the frequency and context of worker–client interactions. Because of the residential context in which articulations of relationship-based work are embedded, there has been an assumption of a relatively high frequency of interaction over defined periods of time. In relational practice, on the other hand, such assumptions are entirely abandoned, and it is equally possible to apply relational practice to one-time encounters as it is to do so to encounters that are intermittently repetitive and unfold over longer periods of time. In this sense, relational practice perhaps more so than relationship-based work lends itself as a framework for child and youth care practice contexts that are nonresidential and do not necessarily unfold within the living context of the child or youth.

PROFESSIONAL ISSUES OF RELATIONSHIPS

It is difficult to separate the professional issues of relationships with those that are clinical, therapeutic or specifically related to how we best address the needs of the clients. Given the centrality of relationships in our work, labeling some issues as professional and others as "not professional" is an artificial construct at best, and in some cases may detract from the complexity of the issue itself. Nevertheless, we will identity a number of issues that reflect the professional context of identity development for child and youth care workers as well as the specific employment context of the worker. To this end, we will explore in some detail three "professional issues" of relationships. First, we will consider the concept of power and how it might influence our approach to relationship-based or relational practice, specifically as it pertains to role definition and questions of authority. Second, we will explore the professional issues entailed in the development of relationships with clients in the context of teams. And third, we will consider the training and professional development context of relationship-based work and relational practice. Before proceeding to exploring these three professional issues, it is important to briefly highlight some language issues that frequently render discussions of relationships confusing.

Language Games with Relationship

Everybody encounters relationships every day, both in their public lives and in their private lives. In fact, we encounter relationships before just about any other social experience in our lives. The mother–child relationship develops in uterus and provides a foundation (albeit a nondeterminative one) for all future relationships. We have certainly learned a lot in recent years about the importance of our early relationships, be that with parents, siblings, or even strangers who might smile at us, caress our cheeks, or, more on the sinister side, behave toward us in abusive ways. We have also learned that what relationships we focus on is related to our developmental stages. As infants we look to parents or principal care givers. As pre-adolescents, we still are focused on our relationships with principal care givers but we start to develop a real interest in peers. By the time we hit adolescence, the peer group really takes over, and the focus of relationships takes on not only social characteristics, but also sexual ones. And as adults, we typically foster relationships with all kinds of different groups, including our own children, our partners, extended families, friends and colleagues (Batsleer, 2008).

Our relationships as adults are not all the same. We intuitively understand that relationships differ in terms of their characteristics, what motivates them and what we do within these relationships. Some relationships exist only due to circumstances. Others are sought out by one, two, or all parties to the relationship. Perhaps most importantly, some relationships bring us joy and happiness while others bring us down and feel like a burden. And in many cases, our relationships are not consistent in terms of how they impact our lives; many relationships have moments of greatness and moments of absolute misery.

The term "relationship" imposes assumptions about its characteristics. The term itself is associated with concepts such as commitment, reliability, trust, and support. There is nothing within the linguistic origins of the term that causes these associations, but there is a great deal in our social constructions of language that contributes to these.

Relationships are constructed as interpersonal connections that are pursued by adults consensually, that remain in place over longer periods of time, that sometimes have some institutional infrastructure to "govern" the relationship (such as marriage), and that constitute "safe zones" for our identities. Within the context of our relationships, we ought to be able to express ourselves freely and in relatively uninhibited ways. And yet when we examine our relationships we quickly realize that not all of them are equal with respect to these socially constructed expectations. In some relationships, only some of these expectations are met, while in others, perhaps none are met.

To some extent, these differences are related to what motivates our relationships in the first place. We typically understand, for example, that our relationships with friends are much more consensual than those with colleagues, especially if we are not that fond of the colleagues or when the colleagues have greater authority in the workplace than us. For many, relationships with their own family differ substantially from the relationships with the in-laws. Similarly, relationships with our own children might differ from those with nephews and nieces or children of our friends. Relationships can be motivated by many different things, but at a minimum we can identify two kinds of motivations: those that are based on the relationship itself and those that require the relationship as a side effect of another relationship or another context.

The first kind of motivation relates to all those relationships that we seek out ourselves and therefore typically include intimate partners, close friends, and in most cases, our own children. This kind of motivation also includes relationships that are inevitable, such as our birth families or our families in which we were raised. Although the experience within all of these kinds of relationships differs considerably from one person to the next, and certainly can involve both positive and negative scenarios and moments, we are generally motivated to be in these relationships because of the relationships themselves; all other motivations are secondary.

The relationships we have at work or with our partners' or our friends' families, on the other hand, are motivated not by those relationships themselves, but rather by their association with other relationships. It is very common, for example, that when a marriage splits up the respective partners either cease or at least reduce their contact with the other partner's family. It is also very common that when a friendship fades, relationships with the friend's family or other social connections also fade. Similarly in the workplace, the relationships we have rarely survive changes in workplaces; one or two might, but most will fade away, notwithstanding our best and often mutually expressed intentions to stay connected. In this way, we quickly realize that our relationships that are motivated not by the relationship itself but by other relationships or other factors such as employment, may not be able to lay claim to concepts such as commitment, reliability and trust in the same way that other, primary relationships can.

One way of expressing the different implications of these two kinds of motivations for relationships is to relate these to the way in which our lives unfold or are lived. Life unfolds *within* our primary relationships and *alongside* our secondary ones. Secondary relationships, like primary ones, are ever present, but it is not the *specific* relationship with this colleague or that in-law that is ever present.

There is, then, also the question about what we actually do in our relationships and how our relationships affect our day-to-day living. We can list many activities that happen in the context of relationships and that are commonly assumed to be symptomatic of relationships. Thus, we talk to each other, we visit each other, we engage in social or recreational activities with each other, we share stories about ourselves with each other, and so on. Again, it becomes clear that there are many variations in terms of what we do within any given relationship that seem to depend primarily on how we interpret the role of the relationship in our lives. It is not at all a given that we would do all of these things in all of our relationships. In many relationships, we might talk to each other but not share anything about each other. In others, we might disclose our innermost secrets to one another and engage in many social or recreational activities together. And again others are based entirely on social and recreational activities but involve very little talking or sharing (teammates on a sports team, for example).

As a result of the multiple relationships we typically maintain in our lives, we are not likely to pursue consistent patterns within any single relationship. In practice, we *do* different things at different times with different people that are connected to us. The intensity of activity within relationships is not specifically connected to the kind of motivation behind the relationship or even the characteristics of that relationship. We might find ourselves disclosing very personal information to someone with whom we have a secondary relationship for business or professional reasons, or we might engage in a recreational activity with a family member or very close friend. What we do in relationships does not entirely capture how we are impacted by specific relationships, because aside from doing things, we are also experiencing our relationships on the level of feelings and thoughts.

It is precisely at the level of feelings and thoughts that relationships really begin to distinguish themselves from one another. Some relationships are enjoyable and associated with fun activities, but they do not necessarily impact our lives beyond the moments we are actively engaged with the other person. Other relationships may not create much fun or enjoyment face-to-face, but they do stay with us long after the physical encounter has ended. These are the relationships that impact our lives the most, because they are with us independently of the physical presence of the other person. We *feel* these relationships on an on-going basis, perhaps more intensely in some moments than in others. And we *think* about these relationships a lot. Sometimes such thoughts are specifically about the other person, and sometimes we are thinking about the relationship itself. Some of the concepts associated with relationships really do come to life in the context of these thoughts and feelings. Commitment or a breach of commitment, reliability or disappointment, trust or betrayal, loyalty or abandonment become preoccupying contemplations, whether they pertain to the other person's actions or our own toward the other person. Within these relationships, the physical space between two people is transcended by a connectivity through the heart, the mind and, one might argue, the soul.

All of these considerations about relationships contribute to the importance of the theme of relationship as a professional issue in child and youth care practice. It is important to reflect on the complexity of the concept of relationship before embarking on a discussion about how this concept creates a wide range of professional issues for the practitioner. This is what we will turn our attention to now.

POWER AND RELATIONSHIP

All relationships are subject to power dynamics, sometimes overtly so and at other times perhaps covertly so. Child and youth care practitioners may well be engaged with children and youth through the medium of relationships, but within that medium there is power and, almost inevitably, the power is distributed unevenly. In other words, all child and youth worker relationships are characterized by power imbalances between the practitioner and the child. Within these power imbalances, the disequilibrium may vary from minimal to oppressive and, in most relationships, aspects of both of these extremes are constantly present (Snow, 2006).

This may be a rather ominous way of starting a discussion about the professional issues entailed in relationships. After all, oppression is not typically one of the sought after outcomes of our work with children and youth. And yet, we do have to acknowledge that we are all familiar with relationships gone bad. Most children and youth we work with are there precisely because of breakdowns in their relationships with family. Most of us either know someone or at least have heard of someone who has experienced violence within their relationship. And surely all of us are all too familiar with issues of child abuse and neglect that arise within the context of familial dynamics and often even in the context of the institutional care structures designed to keep children safe.

This is why it is critically important to understand that relationships do not transcend power imbalances; instead, they are a way of managing such imbalances and of mitigating the worst scenarios that might arise from these. But nothing we do can fully eliminate the potentially destructive impact of some relationships. Much of what contributes to power imbalances in our relationships with children and youth is structurally embedded in institutional dynamics, culture, convention, language, and social expectations.

Institutional Dynamics

Our relationships with children and youth rarely start when we first meet the child. At least for us they rarely start there, because typically someone would have referred the child to us or assigned us to the child. That process already tips the power balance toward us, because with that referral we receive information about the child. By the time we meet the child, she or he knows nothing about us, but we know something, and sometimes a great deal about him, his family, his level of functioning, his medical history, his criminal record, and typically even his behavioral history. In other words, the old adage that "information is power" certainly applies in this context, and when it comes to information, we hold all the power.

Another way in which institutional dynamics set the context for relationships is through the process of agenda setting. We are not typically asked to engage a child or youth just for the fun of it, nor are the children or youth with whom we are to engage selected randomly. Quite to the contrary, the relationships promoted between practitioner and children reflect prior determinations about goals and objectives, methods of interaction, and hoped for outcomes. In other words, by the time we meet the child face-to-face, we already have an agenda whereas the child is typically unclear about what that agenda is and frequently has had no input into developing that agenda. It is perhaps worth noting that many approaches to caring now do include opportunities for the child to be heard (Charlesworth, 2008; Greene, 2005), but this does not in any way mitigate the fact that there is a predetermined agenda in which the child had at best a limited and more often no voice at all. Once we ask the child to have a voice in "something," we have already set the agenda that this "something" ought to take place.

Part of setting an agenda often involves setting a schedule. Institutionally, this process is often determined by available funding, employment law and policies and procedures. Relationships between practitioner and child are not spontaneous but planned within the parameters of the practitioner's work schedule. This too contributes to a power imbalance within the relationship. Related to the issue of scheduling is the issue of case termination. Very often, access to service is time limited, based on program design or funding limitations. Our approach to relationships with children therefore is influenced by our understanding of such time limits. When the time comes, we begin the process of "separation work" whether the child is ready for that or not. In really unfortunate scenarios, separation unfolds because a child reaches a certain age at which he is no longer eligible to receive the services offered, including the service of relationship with the child and youth worker.

Our relationships with children are not private. In and of itself, this changes the nature of relationship from one that is between two parties to one that is wide open in terms of who is party to the relationship. In our private lives, our relationships are private in the sense that there are no formalized requirements about transcending the two person relationship with respect to incorporating input from outside parties or with respect to reporting outputs or outcomes to other parties. We may choose to do so anyway, which can give rise to anything from advice to gossip, but these are private and personal choices. In our relationships with children, on the other hand, inputs are incorporated into the relationship by other professionals, often even a multi-disciplinary team of professionals, as well as sometimes by other family members. And what happens within the relationship with the child is reported not based on the need for advice, but instead, based on predetermined reporting requirements and procedures. In this way, the practitioner and the child are at completely different ends of the power spectrum pertaining to the relationship. While the child can make private and personal choices about what to report to whom and what types of inputs to seek from others, the practitioner must follow institutional requirements and procedures in rendering the relationship public. In this sense, our relationships with children are not interpersonal relationships. They are relationships between a child and a system—or at least an institution—whereby the child often is unaware of the other parties to the relationship.

Perhaps the clearest and most rigid power imbalance within our relationships with children relates to the limitations of "professional" relationships. Such limitations are often articulated as boundary issues, but in fact they are issues of law, risk management, and liability, as well as issues of ethics and morality. It is of course true that the setting of boundaries is not strictly a professional issue but also one that defines the nature of our engagement with the child and therefore one that has considerable influence on the substantive components of the work we do with children. Nevertheless, there are components of boundary setting that are in fact professional issues primarily. These include provisions that prohibit sexual intimacy with children, even where those children are of the legal age of consent. They also include provisions that render it prohibitive to have children join personal family functions, attend to the practitioner's home environment, receive gifts or money from the practitioner, or even enable the practitioner to receive gifts from the child or the child's family. We will discuss the professional implications of these examples. However, for the purpose of this discussion, it is important to recognize the power imbalances contained in all of these provisions. Relationships in our private lives are significant partly because they present us with an infinite range of possibilities and opportunities. The relationships we pursue with children, on the other hand, mitigate this sense of infinite possibilities by imposing limitations that are not negotiable. Whereas in private relationships limitations are imposed by the relationship itself and reflect at least the tacit input of both parties to the relationship, in relationships between practitioner and child, such limitations are imposed by the practitioner alone, typically reflecting institutional requirements as well as professional contemplations about ethics, boundaries, and other factors.

Culture

The institutional dynamics that give rise to power imbalances within practitioner–child relationships unfold within a cultural context that itself creates impetus for power imbalances. It is important to remain conscious that our involvement with children is understood and experienced by the child within this cultural context of power imbalances. If we ask the question "where is power located within our society," we will surely arrive at responses that have been reflective of societal power dynamics for many years and in some cases, centuries. Power is located in gender stereotypes, age, race, and ethnicity. It is also located in factors that are not identity based such as education, access to information, economic class, access to resources, and specific skills, such as language skills. And even beyond such material factors, power is located in social roles as well, of which the most notable in this context is that of the "helper" versus the person or persons in need of help.

The very fact that as professionals, child and youth care practitioners are in the role of the "helper" creates a massive power imbalance that manifests itself most acutely at the beginning of our involvement with a child or a child's family. The concept of "helper" is associated with at least the potential of solutions, whereas the concept of "client" is strongly associated with "problems." In many western cultures, in particular, solutions are much more highly valued than problems, and within cultures that have maintained a strong individualistic paradigm, the idea of personal responsibility even assigns credit for having solutions and blame for having problems. We can readily recognize, then, that the vey assignment of a "client" to a practitioner brings with it a power imbalance that is difficult to transcend.

If we add to this structural imbalance some of the other key spaces where power is located such as gender stereotypes, age or race, we are well on our way to set up the first encounter with a child or family as one that takes place within a deeply entrenched power imbalance that is real and intractable. By way of example, we can imagine a White, male child and youth worker entering, for the first time, the home of an African-Canadian family consisting of a single mother and her daughter who have been struggling with parent–child conflict for some time. If we further imagine a photograph of that initial encounter, capturing the moment of first impressions, we can readily identify where the power in the photograph is located, based not on any of the dynamics between the practitioner and the "clients," but rather based on the cultural manifestations of power dynamics. The first task for the practitioner, therefore, will be to mitigate this power imbalance as the encounter proceeds to the next steps.

There are really endless examples of culturally imposed power imbalances. Gary Weaver (1990) describes the story of a young Native American boy who has to compromise, at least superficially, his ethnic identity in order to gain release from a custody facility. In a residential context, we can imagine a visible minority child and parent coming to the residential program for the first time, perhaps for a pre-admission meeting. All around them are individuals of the visible majority, the pictures on the wall reflect the dominant race and culture, and the management of the organization is primarily male. In addition, notwithstanding the kindness of the child and youth workers receiving this family, it is clear that the child is there because the parent was unable to solve the problem, whereas the child and youth workers at least potentially will solve the problem. The degree of disempowerment that unfolds in such a scenario is rarely articulated, but it clearly is present.

Convention

Yet another way in which power imbalances manifest themselves within the practitioner–client relationship is related to our conventions. This is somewhat distinct from our culture inasmuch as conventions reflect not beliefs and values but rather assumed truths about the right way of doing things. In this sense, conventions are much more closely related to institutional norms and regulations than to culture, but they are still not exactly the same. Our conventions might include such factors as scheduling, meetings, case management procedures, assessments, and diagnoses. More generally, though, our conventions are based on a particular logic of doing what we do, which almost invariably requires some version of the following sequence: identify the problem, work toward a solution, close the case. This sequence produces a wide range of secondary conventions that typically entail information gathering, case planning, case conferencing, intervention design, intervention evaluation, and discharge planning meetings.

In this sense, the way we do things imposes a structure of healing onto children, youth and their families that may or may not correspond to the their particular approach to change or healing. There is, therefore, a fundamental power imbalance in place that requires the "client" to adjust to our conventions with respect to service provision. In a child and youth care context, our work is very much integrated into broader conventions of service provision, and we cannot entirely liberate ourselves from these. When the "client" is assigned to us, we are expected to structure our work according to these conventions. And as we develop relationships with our "clients," this structure of providing service permeates the development of the relationship as well. In fact, the relationship itself is evaluated in accordance with that structure. It is, for example, "conventional" to develop relationships in such a way that they progress from superficial to more meaningful, and that there be very little variation from this progression. When a relationship that had been meaningful appears to be sliding "backwards" to a higher level of superficiality, the evaluation of that relationship might sound the problem alarm. The goal within this framework becomes to restore the meaningful relationship rather than to adjust the work to correspond to the changed nature of the relationship. "Clients" cannot change the course of our fundamental logic of service provision; the end goal must be achieved or the case has to be abandoned.

We can see, then, that convention about how service ought to be delivered, and related expectations about progress, imposes on the "client" a powerful experience that is driven primarily by us rather than by the child or youth. The child's conventions are secondary to those that reflect our expectations of service delivery, even in the context of relationship development.

Language

Language is perhaps the most covert factor within the power imbalance that exists in our relationships with children, youth and their families. We have already discussed some of the language implications of the term "relationship." While we have arrived at a clear distinction between our personal relationships and those we foster within our professional activities, this is not necessarily the case for our "clients." For many, relationship is an undifferentiated concept; one either has a relationship or one does not. Our frequent use of the term relationship, premised as it is on our professional field and knowledge, is not a shared resource with the "client." We hold on to this knowledge at the exclusion of the child, and rather than clarifying the concept of relationship as we perceive it, we express this through the development of boundaries. These boundaries are, most typically, imposed on the child rather than negotiated with the child. Our rationale for doing so ranges from policies and procedures to self care measures to ethics, but none of these rationales are fully exposed to the child.

It is true that we frequently attempt to set our boundaries with the child early into our encounters. This kind of up front approach is designed to restore a sense of honesty and transparency to our relationship work with children, youth and families and, in many respects, it does precisely that. On the other hand, we are hampered in this task by the limitations imposed on us by language; every time we try to explain terms such as relationship to the child, we are very likely going to use terms such boundaries, ethics, and policies and procedures, and these terms too are meaningful to us much more so than to the child. Mitigating some of these language issues requires an enormous effort on our part, as well as a skill level with respect to language deconstruction that is far beyond the training and education of most child and youth care workers.

Language considerations with respect to power imbalances are not limited to the term relationship; in fact, within our relationships with children, a number of core power moves are made on a regular basis. On such move is labeling. Labeling involves giving a name to the things we observe, and this, in turn, involves using language. Once again we are stuck in a language environment that is not necessarily shared with the child. By way of example, consider how we might describe the behavior of a youth who does not follow the rules of the program. In our language, we frequently use the term "struggle" to describe such a situation. From the youth's perspective, however, this term may not capture his frame of mind at all. He might be engaged in a cost-benefit analysis and regularly come to the conclusion that breaking the rules will accrue greater benefits to him than following the rules. In this sense, for the youth there is no struggle at all; his actions are symptomatic of excellent thought process and logical decision-making. Our professional jargon surely provides many examples of such scenarios. Terms such as "taking responsibility," "appropriate" and "inappropriate," "power struggle," and "doing well in the program" are all language outcomes of our professional training and communication styles that impose significant meaning on children and youth without their input or rebuttal.

Our relationships hopefully will develop over time in such a way as to minimize such misunderstandings and mislabeling as presented above. Even when we mitigate some of the language issues inherent in our work, we still have to recognize that language presents a significant power imbalance in our relationships with children, youth, and their families. Ultimately, we control the process by which information about the relationship is externalized through written reports, verbal reports in case conferences, and anecdotal story telling about our "clients." And ultimately we know that the "professional" representation of relationships will carry far more weight in case planning than the informal representation that might come from the "client" directly.

Social Expectations

The power imbalances within our relationships with children, youth and families are highlighted once more in relation to social expectations that are in place for the "client" as service is being received. Perhaps most fundamentally, there is a power imbalance related to choice; after all, once a child and youth worker is assigned a case, the child or family rarely has the opportunity to demand a different worker. In residential programs, child and youth workers are typically assigned as primary workers for specific children or youth admitted to the program, and this process unfolds before any sort of relationship has evolved. In educational settings, special classrooms typically only have one child and youth worker available, and all children within the classroom will have to develop their relationships with that one individual. Child and youth workers assigned to work with families in the family's home similarly are so assigned without prior consultation with the family about the specific characteristics they might value or find more attractive. The relationship will have to be developed with whoever is assigned the case.

The expectation that "clients" work with whoever is assigned is one of many conventions associated with service provision. "Client" expressions of a lack of satisfaction with an assigned worker rarely are taken seriously, and sometimes are even reframed as a "client problem." Beyond this issue of choice, however, social expectations of "client conduct" are, in fact, as extensive if not more so than the social expectations on the practitioner, which further contributes to the power imbalance embedded within the relationship. Since most service provision is publically funded, children and their families are expected to be grateful, or at least to appreciate the services they receive. And since the purpose of service provision is to solve the problems of the "client," he is also expected to "work hard" toward resolving these problems. The judgment as to whether or not she or he is working hard, however, rests entirely with the practitioner. Moreover, the language and methodology of this evaluation comes from within the field of knowledge and expertise associated with the practitioner's professional association, not with the "client's" intuitive or experiential wisdom. In this sense, then, the power imbalance is further accentuated.

RELATIONSHIP DEVELOPMENT IN THE CONTEXT OF TEAMS

Child and youth workers rarely work autonomously. The field itself has developed as a team-based approach to engaging with children and youth. This reflects the dominance of residential care in our history, but even in other employment contexts, team approaches remain central in how the work is done. One of the differences in school-based, hospital-based, or family-centered child and youth care compared to residential care is that teams are not constituted entirely by child and youth workers but typically are multi-disciplinary in nature.

Working as part of a team has many implications for relationship development. Such implications have often been articulated in very positive ways, highlighting the theoretical advantages of working from a team-based approach. According to Krueger (1990, p. 15), for example, "Team members complete the process [of account-ability] by being and holding one another accountable. They strive to be objective observers and to be articulate as they describe their observations of others." Team approaches do present opportunities for great service, but there are many potential issues that emerge and that deserve to be contemplated critically. For one thing, the confidentiality issue is front and centre in this context. In spite of a clear understanding that the relationship between practitioner and child ought to be governed by confidentiality, there is also an understanding that information about children needs to be shared amongst those who also might be engaged with that child. In a residential context, this means that whatever work one practitioner might be doing with a youth must be shared with the other members of the residential team, and often also with external members of that team, such as clinicians and psychiatrists. The professional issue embedded in this is readily apparent. How can we develop a trusting relationship with a child when it is known upfront that the content of the relationship is shared widely with others whom the child may or may not trust or sometimes even know? At the same time, without an understanding that information will be shared within the "team," we may well be doing a disservice to the child, who might assume that his disclosures to one practitioner will result in a united response from all of those involved in his life.

The confidentiality issue entailed in any team-based approach to service provision is symptomatic of the nature of relationships that might evolve in this context. While much of the literature on relationship-based work focuses on the inter-personal relationship between one practitioner and one child, in reality, our relationships with children are not that simple. When we work within a team, the relationships we have with children are much more "porous" than inter-personal relationships. In a sense, these are relationships between a child and a group of people, with one practitioner appointed as spokesperson in the everyday life of the relationship. This is particularly the case in the residential context, given that within that context, the everyday unfolding of relationships is subject to supervision and review of many practitioners. But it typically is also the case in any settings where everyday interaction unfolds in the midst of program operations such as hospitals, schools, and community centers. In some employment contexts, the team might not be as prevalent in its influence on the everyday relationship. Child and youth workers engaged with families in their homes or in outreach capacities, for example, can develop their relationships with the "clients" with much greater autonomy from the team, given that supervision and review of these relationships tend to be much more sporadic.

In addition to issues related to the sharing of information, the practitioner working in the context of a team has to manage several other professional issues that sometimes can be quite challenging. There is, of course, the loyalty issue that comes up frequently. When a child discloses negative experiences or perceptions of another member of the team, the practitioner has to determine an appropriate response. This can range from dismissing the child's perceptions to defending the colleague to attacking the colleague on behalf of the child. In the residential context, this is more often than not resolved in favour of remaining loyal to colleagues rather than the child. The culture of teamwork in residential care is typically very strong, but not always to positive effect, at least from the child's perspective. In nonresidential contexts, team culture can still be very strong, but often it is not quite as dominant a factor in decision-making when it comes to loyalty issues for the practitioner.

One of the challenges associated with teamwork, very much related to the loyalty issue, is that every member of the team could potentially have a relationship with the child. In any employment context where relationship-based work is presented as a requirement, this creates the potential for competition amongst team members for "the best" relationship. In multi-disciplinary teams, practitioner–child relationships vary considerably in nature and scope. For many child and youth care practitioners in particular, the quantity of encounters is often seen as a major criterion in the quality of the relationship. Children, however, rarely substantiate this assumption. Very often, a child might identify a worker who is rarely present as the most important relationship in their lives, which can be frustrating for the child and youth care practitioner who has been face to face with that child every day in multiple settings and contexts.

Finally, the team context of developing relationships also contributes to issues related to boundaries. While the setting of boundaries is primarily a function of the exploration of Self, the team context provides for a rather public context in which such boundaries are set. Deviations from what might be seen as acceptable boundaries are readily identified, and team ideas about consistency and transparency in practitioner–child relationships play a major part in evaluating the appropriateness of particular boundaries set by any given practitioner. In this sense, teams can add limitations to what is possible in terms of relationship development, and such limitations almost always impact on the degree to which relationship-based work really can rely on the exploration of Self as its core ingredient.

RELATIONSHIP TRAINING AND PROFESSIONAL DEVELOPMENT

Relationship-based work is difficult work at the best of times, and the professional issues arising from doing the work in this way are substantial. This raises the question of how to best prepare the practitioner for the work ahead and how to maintain the highest possible quality in this work as the practitioner gains experience and confidence. Given our discussion of power issues entailed in our relationships with children in particular, the importance of ensuring that the practitioner is prepared to mitigate some of these inevitable power dynamics is essential. To some extent, the onus for ensuring adequate training and professional development lies with the employer; after all, managing the professional development regiment of child and youth workers is one very important function of management. On the other hand, the practitioner too has some responsibility in ensuring preparedness for the job. Complacency in this respect is a sure way of limiting the effectiveness of child and youth work and sometimes even of moving into the realm of doing more harm than good.

Training and professional development in child and youth care has been a challenge for some time and across sectors. It has been especially difficult in residential care because of the enormous costs involved in replacing workers on shift to attend training. In nonresidential settings, this replacement cost typically does not apply or at least is more manageable, and therefore the opportunities for training and professional development are significantly enhanced. In residential care, mandatory training required for the purpose of licensing or accreditation does not include any specific focus on relationships. Instead, mandatory training requirements typically include a focus on crisis intervention and physical restraint techniques as well first aid and CPR certification. It is therefore necessary to provide additional opportunities for practitioners to enhance their "relationship skills."

Herein we encounter our first challenge. It is not widely recognized that there is such a thing as "relationship skill." In many practice settings, relationship-based work is mandated by the policies and procedures of the employer, but there are no specific skills articulated to support this mandate. For many employers, most of whom are not themselves professionals within the child and youth care field, relationship development is viewed as an innate skill, one that everyone has to some degree and that is furthered primarily by effort and attention to the prescriptions of policies and procedures. As a result, employers often do not focus their training efforts on the topic of relationships, preferring instead to integrate references to relationship-based work into training events related to myriad other issues and concerns.

As a result of not recognizing that relationship-based work is skill-based work, there is frequently an assumption amongst employers and child and youth care practitioners that having been working in the field and developing relationships with children for many years constitutes confirmation of quality work and high levels of skill. There is no evidentiary basis to make such claim, nor is this a logical claim. Experience in and of itself contributes nothing at all to skill, particularly if that experience has not been evaluated in a reflective and critical manner. Child and youth care workers who have believed themselves to be working through the medium of relationships for many years might have been ignorant of the power issues entailed in their work for all of these years. In that case, one would be hard pressed to refer to their work as skill-based; instead, it more accurately would be described as entrenched oppression, and it would be difficult to change this approach to the work for the better.

This is why it is extremely important that relationship development, and being in relationship with children, youth and families, be a core component of training and professional development for child and youth workers in all settings. Without ongoing attention to these issues, the core principle and operating dynamic of our profession becomes sidelined as an assumed personality trait of those who are currently present in the field. And given the tremendous variations in how people end up working in this field, this is simply not sufficient.

In the absence of relevant training and professional development opportunities initiated by the employer, child and youth care professionals still have a responsibility to improve their skills relevant to relationship-based work. The most important practice that therefore must be integrated into the day to day activities of all child and youth workers is the reflective and reflexive process informed by critical thinking and self-challenge. In some work settings, the supervision process may contribute to this, but in many settings where supervision is either sporadic or focuses primarily on employment related issues and expectations, practitioners must rely on their own commitment to this practice and where possible, on the assistance of their colleagues.

RELATIONAL VERSUS RELATIONSHIP-BASED

In recent years, there has been an increase in the use of the term "relational," sometimes as a synonym for relationship-based work and at other times as a substitute for that term (Garfat, 2008). In closing this discussion about the professional issues arising from our development of relationships with children, youth and families, it is worthwhile to briefly reflect on whether or not the emergence of new thinking pursuant to relational approaches to the work have an impact on the range of professional issues the practitioner might encounter.

The core distinction between the terms "relationship" and "relational" is that the former describes a condition whereas the latter describes a process. It is of course true that relationships unfold over time, and therefore also entail process as a core element of their existence, but fundamentally, at any given point in time, relationships denote a condition. Specifically, they denote the condition of two individuals and their juxtaposition with respect to one another. Relational practice, on the other hand, does not require the condition of relationship to be present at any given moment. This type of practice refers to the dynamics that unfold within the spaces between the Selves, or the physical and emotional identities, of two individuals (Garfat, 2008). In this sense, relational work is much less dependent on the ongoing presence of any specific practitioner. Its focus is more on the experience of any given encounter for both the client and the practitioner(s) involved.

With respect to professional issues, the notion of relational practice holds great promise. The power dynamics entailed in such practice are still present, but they are mitigated by the absence of any material basis of the encounter. All encounters unfold without the weight of previous encounters to consider, which allows for a re-balancing of power imbalances on an on-going and even moment-to-moment basis. Within this construction of "relationship," the concept of relationship is stripped of its potentially oppressive features related to loyalty, commitment and expectations, and re-articulated through its more interactive and momentary features of connectedness and being together in the moment.

This type of approach also mitigates some of the challenges entailed in working through the medium of relationship in the context of teams. New opportunities are presented to the client to experience relational moments with a range of adults and service providers, individually and in groups, without having to determine the implications for each set of interpersonal relationships. In this sense, relational work becomes much more child-centered than relationship-based work, in which clearly the practitioner has as much at stake as the child.

Perhaps the one concern about introducing relational approaches to the field at this time is that these approaches are complex from the practitioner's perspective, and as such, they are even more skill-intensive than relationship-based approaches. In the absence of training and professional development to prepare the practitioner adequately to perform within the relational context, the possibility of missing the point is high.

REFERENCES

Addams, J. (1910). *Twenty years at Hull House*. New York: Macmillan.

Austin, D., & Halpin, W. (1987). Seeing "I" to "I": A phenomenological analysis of the caring relationship. *Journal of Child and Youth Care, 3*(3), 37–42.

Batsleer, J. R. (2008). *Informal learning in youth work*. London: SAGE.

Beck, M., & Malley, J. (1998). A pedagogy of belonging. *Reclaiming Children and Youth, 7*(3), 133–137.

Bendtro, L., Ness, A., & Mitchell, M. (2005). *No disposable kids*. Bloomington, IN: National Education Service.

Bettelheim, B. (1974). *A home for the heart*. New York: Knopf.

Burns, M. (1987). Rapport and relationships as the basis of child care. *Journal of Child and Youth Care, 2*(2), 47–57.

Charlesworth, J. (2008). Inquiry into issues of voice in relational practice. In G. Bellefeuille & F. Ricks (Eds.), *Standing on the precipice: Inquiry into the creative potential of child and youth care practice* (pp. 231–280). Edmonton, Canada: McEwan Press.

Fewster, G. (2001a). Growing together: The personal relationship in child and youth care. *Journal of Child and Youth Care, 15*(4), 5–16

Fewster, G. (2001b). The third person singular: Writing about the child and youth care relationship. *Journal of Child and Youth Care, 15*(4), 77–84.

Garfat, T. (Ed.). (2003). *A child and youth care approach to working with families.* New York: Haworth Press.

Garfat, T. (2008). The inter-personal in-between: An exploration of relational child and youth care practice. In G. Bellefeuille & F. Ricks (Eds.), *Standing on the precipice: Inquiry into the creative potential of child and youth care practice* (pp. 7–34). Edmonton, Canada: McEwan Press.

Gharabaghi, K. (2008). The relationship trap. *CYC OnLine,* 117(November). Retrieved January 31, 2009, from http://www.cyc-net.org/cyc-online/cyconline-nov2008-gharabaghi.html

Greene, R. W. (2005). *The explosive child.* New York: Harper Collins.

Griffin, S. (2008). The spatial environments of street-involved youth: Can the streets be a therapeutic milieu? *Relational Child and Youth Care Practice, 21*(4), 16–27.

Korczak, J. (1992). *When I am little again and the child's right to respect.* New York: University Press of America. (Original work published 1935)

Krueger, M. (1990). Child and youth care organizations. In M. Krueger & N. Powell (Eds.), *Choices in caring* (pp. 1–18). Washington, DC: Child Welfare League of America.

Krueger, M. (2004). *Themes and stories in youth work practice.* New York: The Haworth Press.

Krueger, M. (2007). *Sketching youth, self, and youth work.* Rotterdam: Sense Publishers.

Krueger, M., & Powell, N. (Eds.). (1990). *Choices in caring.* Washington, DC: Child Welfare League of America.

Maier, H. (1992). Rhythmicity: A powerful force for experiencing unity and personal connections. *Journal of Child and Youth Care Work, 8*(7), 7–13.

Parry, P. (1999). Relationships: Thoughts on their origin and their power. *Journal of Child and Youth Care, 13*(2), 9–16.

Shealy, C. (1999). Ask a simple question, get a complex answer: Why "the relationship" in child and youth care is neither "sentimental" nor "bogus." *Journal of Child and Youth Care, 13*(2), 99–124.

Redl, F. (1959). Strategy and technique of the life-space interview. *American Journal of Orthopsychiatry, 29,* 1–18.

Snow, K. (2006). Vulnerable citizens: The oppression of children in care. *Journal of Child and Youth Care Work, 21,* 94–105.

Trieschman, A. E., Whittaker, J., & Bendtro, L. K. (1969). *The other 23 hours: Child care work with emotionally disturbed children in a therapeutic milieu.* Chicago: Aldine Publishers.

Weaver, G. (1990). The crisis of cross-cultural child and youth care. In M. Krueger & N. Powell (Eds.), *Choices in caring* (pp. 54–103). Washington, DC: Child Welfare League of America.

Relationships Within and Outside of the Discipline of Child and Youth Care

SUMMARY. This article explores the practitioner's relationships with colleagues, on teams and with professionals from other disciplines and systems. While there has been much analysis and discussion about relationships between practitioners and clients, there has been relatively little attention paid to the professional relationships that are at the center of the practitioner's day-to-day work. It is within these relationships that practitioners encounter both opportunities and challenges in positioning themselves effectively to deliver a positive service to clients. As such, in this article are descriptions of the relationships amongst child and youth care practitioners, between practitioners and other professionals as well as between practitioners and other systems. Several core themes are identified including the importance of communication and networking as well as the role of power imbalances in defining the nature of such relationships.

KEYWORDS. Interdisciplinary practice, multi-disciplinary practice, networking, professional communication, professional relationships, residential teams, youth-serving systems

While relationship-based practice and relational approaches to child and youth care are frequently discussed in the field's literature, less attention is paid to the relationships between child and youth workers and their peers, other professionals, and other systems (Becker, 2001; Lockhead, 2001; Salhani & Charles, 2007). Yet virtually everything we do as child and youth care professionals involves some level of contact, collaboration, or sometimes conflict with some or all of these groups and systems. Professional issues are perhaps nowhere as clearly present as they are within these relationships. It is therefore important to reflect on the dynamics of such relationships in some detail. Specifically, we will explore the professional issues entailed in our relationships with other child and youth workers, our relationships with professionals from other disciplines, and our relationships with other institutions and systems.

While there have been some excellent discussions of at least many of the professional issues entailed in these relationships, our exploration will take on a different form. Instead of constructing "ideal models" of professional relationships and conduct, we will explore the professional issues both in abstract and in very practical and pragmatic ways. Our effectiveness as a profession is very much impacted by the nature of these relationships, and we simply cannot afford to construct models that cannot be applied in practice settings. The goal of this discussion is to provide the practitioner with an understanding of the issues on the one hand and applied knowledge and skills to mitigate some of these issues on the other hand.

RELATIONSHIPS WITH OTHER CHILD AND YOUTH WORKERS

Professional relationships present a wide range of challenges and opportunities in all contexts; however, it is at times surprising how challenging the relationship *between* child and youth workers can become. There are two distinctive contexts in which child and youth workers develop relationships: They may be working together on a day-to-day basis as a team, as in a residential program or sometimes in a day treatment program, or they may be working together (representing different life spaces) on a project or in relation to a particular child or youth. This scenario is becoming increasingly common because of the increased deployment of child and youth workers in various sectors. It is therefore entirely possible that a case conference about a particular child may feature a child and youth worker from a residential program where the child resides, another from the special education program the child attends, perhaps a child and youth worker supporting the family in some capacity as family worker, and maybe even a child and youth worker from some type of recreational or therapeutic community program.

While there are a number of very specific issues that arise with respect to each of these scenarios that are unique to the scenario, there are some common issues that are worthwhile contemplating at least briefly.

Talking Within the Discipline

When child and youth workers share responsibility for the care of a child or youth, their communication may well reflect differing perspectives. However, they are talking within the general frame of reference of their discipline. Increasingly, therefore, it is possible to have meetings about children where multiple systems and sectors are represented even though the meeting itself is not reflective of a multidisciplinary approach. Multi-sectoral approaches are not at all the same as multi-disciplinary approaches, but each approach has benefits and disadvantages. Within a multi-disciplinary approach unfolding within the same sector (a Children's Mental Health center, for example), the work with a particular child or youth will be influenced by observations and interventions representing multiple perspectives and expertise, including the life space expertise of the child and youth worker, but also the pharmacological and diagnostic expertise of the psychiatrist, the clinical expertise of the psychologist and the learning expertise of the teacher (Nottle & Thompson, 1999; Poulton & West, 1993). Within a multi-sectoral approach managed by a single professional discipline, on the other hand, the work with the child or youth will be influenced by observations and expertise about life spaces (if the discipline is child and youth care) or some other criteria if the discipline is something other than child and youth care.

A multi-disciplinary approach is still limited by the organizational culture of the employer, the particular service model in place and perhaps also by the institutional conventions and policies and procedures governing the process (Guy, 1986; Ho, 1977; Salhani &

Charles, 2007). A multi-sectoral approach, on the other hand, will be limited by the singular perspective brought to bear on understanding the child or youth and developing treatment or intervention plans (Robinson & Cottrell, 2005; Salmon & Rapport, 2005).

As a result of the relationship focus of our discipline, there is the risk that child and youth workers may mistake their respective relationships with the child as an indication of inadequacies in the relationships between the child and child and youth workers from other sectors. Much like child and youth workers from the same team often accuse each other of being too *laissez faire* or too authoritarian within their relationship with a particular child, resulting in behavioral challenges or performance issues for the child, child and youth workers from different sectors may view each other's contribution to the child's experience in similar ways. Thus we often hear a school-based child and youth care worker complaining that the residential child and youth worker is not sufficiently consistent with expectations or the hospital-based child and youth worker complaining about the outreach child and youth worker not being sufficiently vigilant about the child's nutrition.

These kinds of dynamics are reflective of the appearance of competition among like-minded individuals in any context. When multiple child and youth workers representing different sectors become jointly responsible for the care of a child or youth, the risk of the appearance of competitive features in the professional interactions of these workers increases dramatically. Mitigating this risk will require a strong reflective focus on the part of each worker, with an understanding that children experience different life spaces differently, and that therefore, different outcomes or performance levels are to be expected at any given time. This, in turn, will require a strong understanding of roles, and a commitment to avoid getting caught up in perceived hierarchies of child and youth worker roles (Krueger & Stuart, 1999; Ricks & Charlesworth, 1982).

Understanding Roles and Role Hierarchies

Just because a number of individuals in the life of a particular child are child and youth workers does not mean that they all have the same role. The very same dynamics that often result in residential child and youth workers feeling somewhat put out by the apparent power of the counselor or psychologist who sees the child perhaps for one hour per week compared to the residential worker's 24/7 exposure, can unfold in scenarios where the nonresidential professionals are child and youth workers as well. Understanding that even child and youth workers may have limited exposure to a particular child as a result of a specifically delineated role is critical to ensuring constructive relationships between child and youth workers. Amongst child and youth workers, there is an increasing perception that some roles are more prestigious than others. This, in turn, has the potential of resulting in similar patterns of negativity as the disciplinary envy that is sometimes displayed by child and youth workers toward social workers or by social workers toward psychologists (Salhani & Charles, 2007). In child and youth work, a number of job functions and employment settings are often sorted based on perceived prestige and sometimes real differences in compensation with increasing frequency.

Whereas not so long ago residential child and youth care positions were really the only or at least the most prominent positions available, this is no longer the case. With child and youth care professionals employed in hospitals, schools, and other settings and contexts that are nonresidential in nature, the social value associated with some positions becomes a function of criteria that were unfamiliar to the profession in the past. For example, child and youth workers no longer have to accept jobs that require evening and weekend work; they can work nine-to-five jobs Monday through Friday in schools. Similarly, child and youth workers no longer have to accept household management functions as part of their jobs. They can now work within the institutional structures of hospitals, where most such functions fall within the area of responsibility of custodial, kitchen or administrative departments. All of this has resulted in an increased competition for nonresidential positions. It has also resulted in at least the possibility of valuing the roles of some child and youth workers more so than others based on the social prestige of the institutional context of employment. Hospital-based child and youth care is frequently seen as the most prestigious (and potentially therefore the most skill-based) employment context, while residential care increasingly has fallen to the bottom of this hierarchy.

As a discipline, child and youth care is not immune to the cultural ascriptions of value and prestige to different institutions and professional roles. Clearly, such ascriptions fall well outside of the core values of the discipline, but there is no denying that individual practitioners are nevertheless impacted by these and often do not hesitate to apply these to their own peers within the profession. Related to this issue but with a slightly different twist is the issue of our longstanding inferiority complex in relation to other disciplines (Bowie, 2005; Gaughan & Gharabaghi, 1999; Milligan, 1998). Historically, the role of child and youth workers in case management and decision-making about clients has been second to that of social workers, clinical staff, psychologists, or others. In most large organizations, the organizational structure is set up in such a way that decision-making does in fact reflect a disciplinary hierarchy. One consequence of this historical legacy is that child and youth workers often hesitate to make decisions pending approval or endorsement from the social worker or case manager. In situations where child and youth workers are representing the various sectors involved in the life of a particular child, overcoming the need for extra-disciplinary approval will be necessary.

SPECIAL ISSUES FOR RESIDENTIAL TEAMS

The residential context gives rise to a wide range of unique professional issues for child and youth workers. To some extent, child and youth workers working within a residential program are impacted by existing perceptions about their professional status as well as by ongoing dynamics of team work in an intense and frequently crisis-driven environment. There are number of assumptions that are frequently made about residential child and youth workers, most of which are entirely fictitious, but some may actually be at least partially true (Dunlop, 2004; Salhani & Charles, 2007):

- Residential work is a stepping stone to a "real" career in social work;
- Only young and single people can and should do this work;
- The qualifications for doing residential work are a good attitude and a fun-loving personality;
- The real work with children and youth takes place outside of the residential context;
- Residential workers can describe behaviors and potentially useful interventions, but little more than that.

Given these perceptions, residential child and youth worker teams are confronted with the task of ensuring they remain effective in terms of caring for the children and youth in the facility while, at the same time, wanting to change the way in which their professional role is perceived by others. This, in turn, requires an articulation of what they actually do and how what they do corresponds to identifiable functions in the caring for a particular child or group of children. The task does not stop here. Once we have identified what we actually do and what that might look like, we have to first contemplate and then articulate how what we do interfaces with what other professionals do so that our role is not limited but, rather, is recognized as one of several components in the caring for a child (or a group of children/youth).

While individual residential workers can potentially develop their role and establish themselves as valued professionals in the way described, there are additionally the challenges of working on a residential team. In this context, there are benefits and opportunities on the one hand (Durrant, 1993; Fulcher, 1991, 2007; Krueger, 1987), and potential challenges and real dangers on the other hand.

Potential Challenges and Risks of Residential Teams

As much as residential teams can be a source of strength, inspiration and professional growth, there are some inherent risks as well. In many cases, for a variety of reasons, the professional issues emerging out of residential teams reflect some of the less fortunate aspects of child and youth work and often have a very significant impact on the continuous image problems of the profession.

The intensity of residential work often gives rise to a loss of boundaries between staff members. As a residential worker, the day-to-day tasks are not dissimilar to household management in many respects, and many child and youth workers find themselves struggling with maintaining the professional purpose of household management separate from the closeness or sometimes conflict that can emerge when jointly trying to manage the affairs of day-to-day life. Personal relationships, cliques, gossip, and mistrust are all too frequently mainstays of residential teams. Children and youth are very perceptive in this regard, and it is almost never possible to keep them from feeling the impact of this kind of team dysfunction. Discord and conflict, negativity and dissatisfaction have a way of spreading through any social context, and the residents are not immune to this.

Similarly, the informality associated with doing residential work can at times lead to an abandonment of professional conduct. On the one hand, there is good reason to maintain an informal and relatively casual approach to one's choices in clothing, use of language, speed of task completion, and sense of humor. On the other hand, it is the strategic, thoughtful, and planned use of informality that serves a constructive purpose in residential work. On many teams, this part is simply forgotten, and child and youth workers begin to behave in ways they might in their social lives with their own peers. The result is inappropriate dress, poor role modeling with respect to self-care and presentation, edgy use of language or, alternatively, an excessive use of adult-based humor. Sometimes it is not the adult content of the humor that is problematic but the humorous references to the personal lives of staff, otherwise known as "inside jokes"; the consequence is making other residents and colleagues feel left out.

Perhaps most distressing is the emergence of a sense of ownership and entitlement on the part of many residential teams. When residents report disliking what they perceive as an "us versus them mentality" on the part of the staff, they are typically quite accurate in their analysis of the situation. Many staff teams develop a misguided sense of ownership over the living environment and begin to hold residents accountable for having an impact on their own living environment by, for example, redecorating, expressing dislike of certain physical features in the home, or by putting their feet on the coffee table (something that is almost always done by staff during team meetings held in the residence's living room). Even within the team, conflict can emerge based on workers' sense of ownership status over the physical environment. Invariably, there are some workers who take on the role of household manager with greater enthusiasm and determination than others, and before long, informal rules about who is in charge are established. The tension between doing residential work and administering a residential program is quite prevalent throughout this sector and typically manifests itself through office sitting. When residential staff begin to execute their child and youth work while sitting in the staff office, the team has legitimized the abandonment of doing residential work and the adoption of administering a program in which residents are by and large seen as subjects to comply (Gharabaghi, 2008).

Finally, there is the issue of loyalty and accountability within residential teams. In theory, accountability should be furthered by virtue of the presence of team: more people see what you do and comment on it. In practice, however, this is not always the case (Salhani & Charles, 2007). Residential child and youth workers are constantly confronted with the issue of loyalty to their colleagues versus fairness to the residents. Excellent team work is in fact often articulated as including unity, togetherness, staff backing each other up, consistency, trust and loyalty. The implications of this articulation of team work include barriers to honest feedback, the disempowerment of residents, and a slim likelihood that the voice of residents is not only heard, but in fact encouraged and nurtured.

RELATIONSHIPS WITH OTHER PROFESSIONALS

Some of the most important relationships child and youth workers develop are with other professionals. One of the reasons these relationships are so important is because it is in the context of our interactions with professionals from a wide range of disciplines that the substance of our work with children, youth, and families becomes meaningful within the broader context of case management and decision-making. Yet this is also an area in which child and youth workers have encountered many challenges. Frequently one hears the complaint from child and youth workers that their voice is dismissed or simply not taken seriously in the context of case conferences, the development of a plan of care or discussions about the particular directions an intervention is to take. Residential child and youth workers in particular often find this enormously frustrating because it is they who spend the majority of time with the children or youth. How can someone who only sees the child or youth for an hour each week have so much more influence in case management or in decision-making? Partly in response to this dilemma, Trieschman, Brendtro, and Whittaker (1969) wrote their now very famous book, *The Other 23 Hours*. In it they delineate very clearly the importance of the day-to-day work related to guiding children and youth through the process of living, growing, and learning. They also point to the important role of other professionals, even if those only have limited or sporadic contact with the children or youth.

It is important to think about why child and youth workers are not always taken as seriously as they would like in multi-disciplinary approaches to working with children, youth or families. Perhaps one reason relates to the lack of understanding other professionals have of the role of child and youth workers. Then again, perhaps we need to ask whose responsibility it really is to ensure that everyone involved understands the role. One possible answer is that child and youth workers themselves have not always done particularly well in articulating what it is they do and how it relates to what others are doing. There is no doubt that the language used to provide a framework for understanding the work of different professionals is significantly underdeveloped amongst child and youth workers generally.

One of the challenges of the multi-disciplinary process and of the involvement of so many sectors and professionals in the lives of children, youth and families is that each of these sectors comes with its own set of assumptions and values and typically very distinctive rules and processes that often are not very flexible (Darlington, Feeney, & Rixon, 2005; Gilbert et al., 2000; Mitchener & Field, 1998). In addition, each professional representing a particular sector will do so by speaking the language of their service sector. As child and youth workers we have to therefore develop the capacity to understand all of these languages, to be familiar with the subtext of sector-specific expressions and concepts and to interface each of the sectoral languages with the language and culture of child and youth work.

We can quickly identify a number of fairly concrete professional issues that emerge from this scenario.

- In order to be able to effectively communicate with all of these professionals, child and youth workers must have an understanding of the roles of these professionals from the perspective of the sectors which these professionals represent. A very common reason for frustration and friction in the relationships between child and youth workers and other professionals is simply a lack of understanding of what these individuals' roles really are.
- In order to be able to relay their information to these other professionals, child and youth workers must develop the capacity to articulate their work in such a way that it transcends a simple description of client behaviors or a sequential account of the child and youth worker's activities.

• Many of the professionals with whom child and youth workers interact represent a problem-focused approach to the client, not so much because this represents the values of their professions but, rather, because their specific roles tend to relate to identified problems or concerns in the behaviors or experiences of the client. Child and youth workers, in contrast, have a responsibility to think of the whole person or family system and therefore ensure that there is balance between deficit areas and strengths. In addition, child and youth workers seek to empower clients to gain strength and to experience growth on their terms, which is often not a shared goal of other professions.

It is becoming quite apparent that in terms of relationships with other professionals, one of the key areas of focus for the child and youth worker discipline is communication and reporting skills (Casson, 2005). One of the key concepts entailed in such a focus is the concept of language. Language is, of course, the basis of all communication. The issue here is not only the accuracy of grammar and the depth of vocabulary but also the fluency of the language and what it is able to cover. Fluency denotes the ability to describe and give meaning to specific observations using the core principles of child and youth work. Coverage denotes the ability to transcend the description of behaviors and to focus instead on experiences and interactions within relationships. Where child and youth workers demonstrate hesitancy in the articulation of their work, much of their perspective is likely to get lost in the either clinical or the often exceedingly concrete worlds of other disciplines. With no clear voice, the child and youth work perspective loses priority on the agenda, and the opportunity for advocacy on behalf of a child, youth, or family can easily be lost.

One of the areas in which the language of child and youth care can play a major role is diversity. Consideration of identity issues is very often neglected or sidelined in the multi-disciplinary case management or treatment processes. One reason for this is that most professionals at the table are focused on *a priori* identified problem or growth areas of the client; whether this relates to the medication regime of the child or her or his academic progress, the knowledge and related strategies that form the foundation of ongoing intervention are typically taken from the evidence base of the research literature, which touts itself as having universal applicability. Yet we all know that each individual is in fact quite unique and that it is generally not at all a good idea to make assumptions about children or families that are based on social patterns or large sample observations.

It is very likely that many cultural contexts will experience the multi-disciplinary process as quite problematic and will likely find the language of that process and the input from many of its components quite challenging to incorporate into lifestyles. The medical establishment, educators, and the criminal justice system, along with all other larger bureaucratic systems, generally do not base their approaches to clients on the latter's life spaces. As such, it is the clients that have to adapt to the needs of those systems rather than the systems trying to understand and engage with specific identities.

Identity is of course not only a matter of culture or ethnicity. Issues of sexual orientation, socio-economic status, mental and emotional health, and so forth, also interface with the physical context of an individual's life and thus impact on the capacity of individuals to function or produce in line with the quasi-scientific expectation of professions that are disconnected from the everyday living of the client. One of the major contributions a child and youth worker can therefore make in the context of the multi-disciplinary case management or treatment process is to ensure that diversity considerations are included in all aspects of assessment and decision-making (VanderVen, 1991). Once again, language is key: It is not only a matter of considering identity descriptors but also of assessing and elaborating on how these impact on a client's relationships with other professionals, peers, the community, institutions, and so forth.

Power Dynamics within Inter-Professional Relationships

Power dynamics are essentially always involved in human interaction, and this is no different in the context of a child and youth worker's relationships with other professionals (Salhani & Charles, 2007). In spite of the extensive knowledge a child and youth worker typically has of a client, there are pre-existing power dynamics that are not easily adjusted or addressed. Historically, child and youth workers have been seen and perhaps saw themselves as less important and less valuable than many other professions (Charles & Gabor, 1991; Gaughan & Gharabaghi, 2008). Those representing the medical establishment, for example, are typically given far more weight in case consultations, case conferences, and multi-disciplinary treatment approaches than are child and youth workers. The social understanding of and respect for sectors such as health care, justice, and education can be quite intimidating given the lack of understanding often displayed toward the child and youth work discipline and settings where child and youth workers feature prominently.

The power dynamic is further entrenched as a result of the legislative context in which specific professionals are involved with client. As probation workers, doctors, and educators frame their roles *vis-à-vis* the client in terms of legislative requirements and the rules of bureaucratic processes, their input into decision-making is anticipated much more so than that of child and youth workers whose role is not always connected to a mandated legislative requirement. In this sense, child and youth workers involved in multi-disciplinary processes do not have ultimate decision-making authority over any aspect of the case, which sets them somewhat apart from a power perspective from the colleagues from other disciplines.

Finally, still in the context of power, we also have to take account of dominant paradigms and value systems in the assessment and treatment of clients. The medical model, social deficit and behavioral models, or any range of accountability models still feature far more prominently amongst the helping professions than does relational work as articulated within the child and youth work discipline. As a result, the power differential between child and youth workers and other professionals is at least in part perpetuated by the ongoing hegemony of a particular paradigm.

None of this implies that child and youth care practitioners should simply surrender to these power dynamics. To the contrary, so long as we recognize the professional issues entailed in our relationship with other professionals, we can take steps to bolster our own confidence in multi-disciplinary processes. As suggested, the most important step we can take is focusing our energy on developing the language skills to participate actively and substantially in multi-disciplinary discussions and case management processes.

Relationships with Other Systems

Given the focus on life spaces in child and youth work, it is nearly impossible and certainly not desirable to avoid contact and connections with the other systems involved with the children, youth, or families to whom we are connected. Whether our role is to assist a client in navigating such systems, advocating to other systems on behalf of our client or, perhaps, supporting other systems in managing our client, as child and youth workers we will almost certainly be interacting with a wide range of systems and the institutions that give life to those systems. Perhaps the most common ones are systems and their institutions that themselves rely quite heavily on the child and youth work discipline in their day-to-day operations. Some obvious ones would include education, health care, child welfare and youth justice. All of these systems have in common a substantial and often cumbersome bureaucracy featuring rules for access and rationales for exclusion as well as regulating the processes of decision-making, appeal, and consultation. In all cases, the institutions within these systems tend to be very hierarchically organized with only the most upper levels of management being able to overturn routine process in the face of extraordinary situations.

One result of the bureaucratic nature of these systems and institutions is that it becomes very difficult and often very frustrating to navigate these with or on behalf of a client. Since child and youth worker involvement with a child, youth, or family almost always implies an "extraordinary" situation, the hierarchical nature of decision-making means that it is very difficult to make progress in any efforts to advance the interests of a client or to provide opportunities for clients that may require the system or institution to give the client the benefit of the doubt. What is required, then, is a solid plan or strategy for child and youth workers to approach the task of getting involved with or connected to other systems and institutions. Let us explore what some of the components of such plan might look like.

Networking, Prior Connections and Relationships

Child and youth workers often do not think about concepts such as networking and making connections with others in the field unless there is a common interest in a client. Somehow, these concepts are associated with the world of business, and there usually are reasons why individuals choose to be child and youth workers; a dislike of business processes and culture is often one of the reasons. It is time to reflect on this a little. As it turns out, there is great benefit to networking and establishing connections even in the absence of common clients at any given time. The most effective way of breaking down the barriers imposed by highly bureaucratic systems and institutional organization often is using personal and professional networks and connections to people on the inside.

This is not a matter of circumventing or breaking the rules. Instead, this is about understanding that in any bureaucracy there are ways of accelerating process and ways of prioritizing files, issues or agenda items that are typically known only to those who are inside of the bureaucracy. Often a particular process changes or is adjusted but no one outside of the daily users of that process may know about this adjustment. Often there is in fact a way of bypassing one or several steps to reach the decision-makers, but understanding the process by which this is possible may not be so easy. Quite frequently and, perhaps surprisingly, the specific order in which issues are being considered and worked on is quite arbitrary and there are no rules about bringing a particular task or issue to the attention of someone so that it is worked on earlier rather than later. That, in turn, is best accomplished through individuals directly connected to that work and with regular access to the workers involved.

By way of preparing for the need to navigate a wide range of systems and institutions, therefore, child and youth workers would be very well advised to consider networking and making connections in other institutions as an integral part of their role. Chances are very high that these contacts will be beneficial to the child and youth worker and, by extension, to a child, youth, or family sometime down the road. Networking, notwithstanding its reputation as a shallow process within the business world, is a significant professional skill that requires good organization and a strong habit of following up with individuals and organizations. As a professional issue, networking in child and youth care presents an obligation that is full of opportunity. Activities that relate to networking are highly compatible with several other professional issues and obligations, including keeping up with best practices in the field (an ethical obligation for the practitioner). This can be done by attending conferences and professional learning opportunities where one is almost certain to meet professionals from other systems and institutions. It can also be done by becoming a member in associations and learning or practice networks.

Beyond the initial encounter of individuals representing a range of systems, child and youth workers ought to be particularly well equipped with maintaining such connections through the medium of ongoing relationships. In many respects, this process requires the same focus on relationship-based work or relational approaches than our work with children. While the relationship itself might be quite different, the focus on connections remains central.

Understanding How Other Systems and Institutions Work

Notwithstanding the benefits of knowing people in other systems and institutions, it is still very important to have a relatively strong and up-to-date understanding of how these other systems and institutions function. This means focusing on how they are organized, how decisions are typically made, and what the goals and objectives are. By doing so, we might also gain a better understanding of the limitations of other systems, which may assist us in contributing to solution-focused discussions when advocating on behalf of clients.

Child and youth workers often underestimate the importance of staying current in their knowledge of processes, systems, institutional structures, and regulation pertaining to people and places other than their daily workplace. Often they are not even all that interested in the organizational structure of their own discipline. Yet understanding one's role, as well as the possibilities and opportunities that are embedded in that role, is to a significant degree a function of understanding everyone else's role and the contexts in which those roles unfold.

Communication and Language

Any professional is judged not only by what she or he does but also (and often more so) by how she or he articulates what she or he does. The ability to convey useful information is critical for successfully engaging with bureaucracies anywhere. Child and youth workers have to remain conscious of this simple fact of professional life, particularly given that the work we do often does not lend itself for clear articulation. The concept of conveying useful information is a difficult one. What exactly does this mean? What might be seen as useful by the child and youth care practitioner may or may not be seen as useful by someone else. As a result of the inherently subjective nature of this dynamic, it helps to know how other institutions use and interpret information to fit their institutional context. This allows the practitioner to provide input into a multi-sectoral and multi-disciplinary case discussion that is not only "heard" but in fact absorbed into the evolution of the case.

Language is the core ingredient in our interactions with other institutions. Deconstructing our language even minimally reveals some major use of jargon as well as terminology that either invokes profoundly different images than what we might have intended or otherwise significantly pathologizes the children and youth we work with. We can consider, for example, the use of the term "to struggle." Child and youth workers frequently use this term to describe a youth's difficulties with following the rules and/or routines of the program, be that a residential program or any other sort of day or evening program. Yet what is meant to be a simple descriptor in fact constitutes a loaded scenario in which the use of jargon could really reduce the opportunities of a youth. The term struggle has potential implications about capacity (as in "he is trying his best but he just cannot keep up"), about motivation (as in "he is lazy, just not trying hard enough, he is stubborn"), and about an *a priori* determination about what is right and what is wrong (which implies a rejection of the youth's perspective before it is even articulated). Furthermore, there are unspoken implications about the philosophy of the program itself. Note that we almost never say that the program struggles with serving this youth effectively; it is typically the youth who struggles with adapting to the demands of the program. There is an unspoken requirement for the youth to assimilate into the program rather than for the program to find ways of serving the youth in the context of his or her unique characteristics and personality traits.

It is extremely important to choose our language carefully and to ensure that we are in fact relaying the information and thoughts that we intended to relay. As we make efforts to adjust our language and the choice of information to the individuals, disciplines and sectors we are working with it is, of course, equally important to ensure that those individuals, disciplines and sectors retain the value of what we bring. One of the longstanding professional issues encountered by child and youth workers in multi-disciplinary settings and in a multi-sectoral context is that of credibility. We have already discussed one side of raising our credibility: Choosing what information we relay and how we articulate it is critically important. But credibility goes beyond supplying information. We too have a vested interest in incorporating the information from others into our work. In order to enhance our credibility, we have to be recognized not only as suppliers of information but also as individuals/professionals who can receive information from others, translate that information into our day-to-day work and add value to the work of others by doing so.

The role of the child and youth worker can increase exponentially when other professionals figure out that this role can give their expertise relevance on a day-to-day basis. Many of the other institutions our clients might be involved with have access to our clients only while they are present at an appointment (health care, counseling), during the school day (schools, day programs), at an individual session (child welfare workers, children's mental health clinicians, probation workers), or during major crises (emergency rooms, police, Intake child welfare workers). Once these institutions recognize that as child and youth workers we could bring their concerns to bear on the client 24 hours per day and in the context of wherever the client may live, work, or play, child and youth workers suddenly receive special invitations to meetings and become major contributors to how a case evolves.

Credibility, of course, does not come with criticizing other institutions for not recognizing what ought to be fairly obvious but, instead, it comes from effectively conveying these possibilities through our work and the language we use to describe our work on an ongoing basis.

Other Systems as Life Spaces

The temptation to engage in battle with systems and bureaucracies on behalf of a child, youth, or family is often great. The personal and intimate contact with a client always appears so much more compelling than the impersonal and technocratic functioning of bureaucracy. Without a doubt, there are times when we do have to take on the role of advocate and challenge the decisions or even the process of institutions. More commonly, however, we have to maintain a consistent view of our own involvement with our clients. From a child and youth work perspective, these other institutions are some of the life spaces of our clients. We engage with these institutions as systems of service. Our clients are connected to these institutions directly through their own life experiences. Rather than fighting with these institutions, we have to ensure that we remain child-centered and that our interests remain focused on our clients' interaction and connection to them, no matter what form this might take.

We also have to ensure that we maintain some perspective on outcomes. On the one hand, one would certainly view outcomes as important: Is the child successful in school? Did she or he avoid being sent to custody? Is she or he safe and cared for? On the other hand, whereas many professions place significant priority on evaluating such outcomes and typically associate time frames with achieving these outcomes, from a child and youth work perspective outcomes are secondary to the experience of our clients as they are connecting with various systems. In the end, any expectation that a connection with one of the major systems or bureaucracies will produce a definitive outcome or will negate further system involvement belies both the complexity and also the purpose of our role with respect to the child, youth, or family. The goal, after all, is not for us to alter the life spaces of our clients but rather to enhance their capacity to manage themselves within their life spaces and to make alterations to those spaces in their time, their way, and their language. For this reason, we remain primarily interested in the way in which our clients experience their involvement with any given system and we explore with them and the system how their actions and procedures might be impacting on these experiences.

REFERENCES

Beker, J. (2001). Development of a professional identity for the child and youth care worker. *Child and Youth Care Forum, 30*(6), 345–354.

Bowie, V. (2005). Youthwork education: A view from down under. *Child and Youth Care Forum, 34*(4), 279–302.

Charles, G., & Gabor, P. (1991). An historical perspective of residential services for troubled and troubling young people in Canada. In G. Charles & S. McIntyre (Eds.), *The best in care: Recommendations for the future of residential services for troubled young people in Canada* (pp. 7–22). Ottawa, Canada: Canadian Child Welfare Association.

Casson, S. F. (2005). Developing a shared language and practice. *Child and Youth Services, 27,* 117–149.

Darlington, Y., Feeney, J. A., & Rixon, K. (2005). Interagency collaboration between child protection and mental health services: Practices, attitudes and barriers. *Child Abuse & Neglect, 29*(10), 1085–1098.

Dunlop, T. (2004). Framing a new and expanded vision for the future of child and youth care work: An international, intercultural and trans-disciplinary perspective. *Journal of Child and Youth Care Work, 19,* 254–267.

Durrant, M. (1993). *Residential treatment: A cooperative, competency-based approach to therapy and program design.* New York: Norton & Company.

Fulcher, L. (1991). Teamwork in residential care. In J. Beker & Z. Eisikovits (Eds.), *Knowledge utilization in residential child and youth care practice* (pp. 215–235). Washington, DC: Child Welfare League of America.

Fulcher, L. (2007). Residential child and youth care is fundamentally about team work. *Relational Child and Youth Care Practice, 20*(4), 30–36.

Gaughan, P., & Gharabaghi, K. (1999). The prospects and dilemmas of child and youth work as a professional discipline. *Journal of Child and Youth Care, 13*(1), 1–18.

Gharabaghi, K. (2008). A quiet cancer: Reflections on the office space in residential care. *CYC OnLine*, 110. Retrieved January 31, 2009, from http://www.cyc-net. org/cyc-online/cycol-0408-gharabaghi.html

Gilbert, J. V., Camp, R. D., Cole, C. D., Bruce, C., Fielding, D. W., & Stanton, S .J. (2001). Preparing students for interpersonal teamwork in healthcare. *Journal of Interprofessional Care, 14*(3), 223–235.

Guy, M. (1986). Interdisciplinary conflict and organizational complexity. *Hospital and Health Sciences Adminstration, 31*, 110–121.

Ho, M. (1977). An analysis of the dynamics of interdisciplinary collaboration. *Child Care Quarterly, 6*, 279–287.

Krueger, M. (1987). Making the team approach work in residential group care. *Child Welfare, 66*, 447–457.

Krueger, M., & Stuart, C. (1999). Context and competence in work with children and youth. *Child and Youth Care Forum, 28*(3), 195–204.

Lochhead, A. (2001). Reflecting on professionalization in child and youth care. *Child and Youth Care Forum, 30*(2), 73–82.

Milligan, I. (1998). Residential child care is not social work! *Social Work Education, 17*(3), 275–285.

Mitchener, C. P., & Fields, K. (1998). Identity and boundary tensions when educators and mental health professionals collaborate between wish and reality. *Child and Adolescent Social Work Journal, 15*(6), 497–512.

Nottle, C., & Thompson, D. J. (1999). Organizations and effectiveness of multi-disciplinary pediatric teams: A pilot survey of three teams. *Physiotherapy, 85*(4), 181–187.

Poulton, B. C., & West, M. (1993). Effective multidisciplinary team work in primary health care. *Journal of Advanced Nursing, 18*, 918–925.

Ricks, F., & Charlesworth, J. (1982). Role and function of child care workers. *Journal of Child and Youth Care, 1*(1), 35–44.

Robinson, M., & Cottrell, D. (2005). Health professionals in multi-disciplinary and multi-agency teams: Changing professional practice. *Journal of Interprofessional Care, 19*(6), 547–560.

Salhani, D., & Charles, G. (2007). The dynamics of an inter-professional team: The interplay of child and youth care with other professions within a residential treatment milieu. *Relational Child and Youth Care Practice, 20*(4), 12–20.

Salmon, G., & Rapport, F. (2005). Multi-agency voices: A thematic analysis of multi-agency working practices within the setting of a child and adolescent mental health service. *Journal of Interprofessional Care, 19*(5), 429–443.

Trieschman, A. E., Whittaker, A., & Bendtro, L. (1969). *The other 23 hours: Child care work with emotionally disturbed children in a therapeutic milieu.* New York: Aldine de Gruyter.

VanderVen, K. (1991). How is child and youth care unique—and different—from other fields? Reflections in time, space and context, with thanks to Albert Einstein. *Journal of Child and Youth Care, 5*(1), 15–19.

The Community Context of Child and Youth Care Practice

SUMMARY. Child and youth care practice unfolds within the context of the community. It is therefore essential that practitioners develop reflective skills not only in relation to their clients and the organizational context in which they are employed, but also in relation to their presence within a community and the community's perception of the practitioner's presence. The role of community within child and youth care practice is explored in relation to the professional issues that can arise for practitioners. It is argued that practitioners both use and contribute to the communities in which they work and that, therefore, an active engagement with communities will require the practitioner to be aware of the implications of their presence with respect to culture, power and community conventions. Finally, the possibility of expanding the role of the practitioner to incorporate community capacity building is also explored. Child and youth care practice is ideally situated to contribute proactively to community capacity as in most communities, capacity issues are very much related to living with children and youth.

KEYWORDS. Child and youth care practice, community-based services, community capacity building, community engagement, community services, culture, diversity, power, families, youth

Child and youth care practice unfolds within the context of communities. This may appear as a fairly obvious statement. However, it is not one that our profession can claim to have consistently incorporated into day-to-day activities. The relative absence of thinking and acting within the context of community within our profession constitutes a significant professional issue in and of itself. Even where child and youth worker roles involve regular contact and interaction with the community, there often is minimal discussion or reflective thought invested in these. In this sense, the profession has failed to keep up with trends in many of the child and youth serving sectors. Over the course of the past twenty years, child protection, children's mental health and even youth justice initiatives have been repeatedly criticized for their institutional focus and their perceived inaccessibility to various communities and social groups. Entire models of alternative approaches to service delivery that are integrated into community development and community capacity building frameworks have been designed, proposed and ultimately not implemented, at least not to the extent that the proponents of such frameworks would like to see. Within the discipline of child and youth care, the role of community has only slowly made it to the broader agenda of service delivery, although there have been some very strong voices advocating for child and youth care approaches that are more fully integrated into an understanding and engagement of communities (Barter, 2003; Mannes, Roehlkepartain, & Benson, 2005).

Much research has shown that the integration of community and children's everyday experiences results in significant improvements in terms of child (and youth) well being. The Search Institute's 40 asset model, the resiliency research produced by the International Resilience Project and even more scientifically-premised research related to brain development have all concluded that community represents a major factor in the lives of healthy and productive children and youth (Kovner Kline, 2008; Scales et al., 2001; Ungar, 2005).

It is important to distinguish between terms such as community involvement and community engagement on the one hand and community-based activities on the other. Taking children and youth into the community to engage in specific activities has been a major component of child and youth care practice for as long as there have been child and youth workers (Banks, 1993; Smale, 1995). For many practitioners, community activities are considered the best part of the job. Children and youth tend to have fun and usually tend to be engaged in whatever the activity might be, and child and youth workers get to participate in activities to which they may not normally have access. Community-based activities do not, however, require any kind of community involvement or engagement. In fact, more often than not, such activities involve simply transferring the program (group home, after-school program, or even family unit for in-home support programs) physically to a community-based location. Many such activities unfold without any contact with community members. Taking a group of children or youth to the movies, for example, may well qualify as a community-based activity, but it is not an activity that requires community involvement outside of access to the theatre or community engagement outside of paying for the tickets.

WHAT IS COMMUNITY?

For many child and youth care practitioners, the concept of community is often equated with the concept of neighborhood, probably because of the long standing association between the discipline of child and youth care and residential care. The "community-based" group home emerged in larger numbers during the 1970s and by the end of the 20th century constituted the norm in terms of residential service delivery in most sectors. "Community-based" in this context typically meant the operation of a group home in a neighborhood instead of on campus-like grounds or inside of larger institutional buildings. Such programs were deemed "community-based" by virtue of their physical appearance as "normal" family homes and their physical location in "normal" neighborhoods. On a day-to-day basis, these group homes encountered the neighborhood through the momentary interactions with neighbors who sometimes condemned and resented the group home's presence.

Community is not, however, just another word for neighborhood (McKnight, 1995). In fact, whereas neighborhoods are defined on the basis of identifiable geographic spaces, typically limited to a few streets and possibly a neighborhood park, a school, and maybe a recreation center, communities may or may not be constituted through contiguous geographic spaces. We might refer to a particular part of town as a community, in which case we would include all the residents, the businesses and the social and cultural services and activities as forming a part of that community. Some such geographic communities may be characterized by high concentrations of particular social identities such as an ethnic group or a gay community or commonalities of economic status. Others might be characterized by very high levels of diversity with many ethnicities, a wide range of economic statuses, and multiple other social identities all living together in a particular geographic space.

Communities do not have to be characterized by geographic contiguity. Some communities are identified based on specific cultural or other identity factors and such communities might live dispersed across a larger city and beyond. The main criterion for identifying such a community is the self-identification of membership. The concept of self-identification is an important aspect of thinking about community. In many cases, communities are defined by others for a group of people, which is the first step in community disempowerment. Particularly in the context of youth, community self-identification may clash significantly with the imposed identifications of community belonging. Youth gangs, for example, may well be characterized as a form of community by member youth but are typically rejected as such by adults. Similarly, while parents may impose on their children identification with a particular cultural or religious community, the children may not accept such identifications and rebel against them.

Another important aspect of communities is that most are not neatly separated from other communities, and individual members within communities most often self-identify as members of multiple communities simultaneously. In other words, most communities are porous and overlap with other communities in substantial ways. Any given person might identify as a member of the Latino community within the context of a large urban area as well as a member of Jewish community globally and a particular professional community locally, nationally or globally.

Although community and neighborhood are not equivalent concepts, neighborhoods nevertheless are important in the context of thinking about community, particularly in the child and youth care context. Neighborhoods more so than communities are where people live; there may or may not be resources within the neighborhood that contribute to the everyday life of the residents, but the experience of that everyday life nevertheless unfolds within the relatively narrow context of one's neighborhood. This is particularly the case for children and youth, who often lack the resources to spend their everyday lives too far from home. Understanding the everyday lives of children, youth, and families therefore requires an understanding of the self-identifications with respect to community and the dynamics within the neighborhood.

From a child and youth care perspective, the importance of neighborhoods and communities cannot possibly be overstated. Given the focus within the discipline on life spaces, the experiences of children and youth within their life spaces cannot be understood outside of the neighborhood and community context (McElwee, 2007; Pittman, 2000). Moreover, a great deal of research focused on issues of resilience and healthy development has focused on the roles of community factors and virtually always has concluded that children and youth will experience healthier and more productive outcomes when surrounded by community support and guidance (Barter, 2004; Mannes et al., 2005). This would seem to indicate that child and youth worker involvement in the community and the neighborhood is an essential component of child and youth care practice. One way of determining whether or not a practitioner has incorporated community in her thinking and reflecting is to ask her for the names of the neighbors. Whether engaged with children, youth, or families in a residential context or in the family home, how many practitioners could answer that question?

REASONS FOR COMMUNITY ENGAGEMENT

Child and youth workers try to find ways of incorporating children, youth, and families in community-based activities, or, alternatively, they are doing damage control and seeking forgiveness from community services for damages or negative experiences with their clients (most commonly youth). In this respect, the engagement with the community is frequently *reactive*. An alternative way of thinking about community and child and youth work is to take a much more *proactive* approach in which child and youth workers seek to make connections with the community that mirror those the practitioner develops with children, youth or families. Before pursuing this further, it is important to explore in greater detail some of the reasons why child and youth care practitioners might be interested in incorporating community engagement and maybe even community capacity building into the discipline and their day-to-day professional activities.

In forming relationships with the community, we can consider a range of scenarios that might become relevant. Three fairly obvious ones are as follows:

- Child and youth workers seeking to find service for a specific client or client group;
- Child and youth workers responding to community complaints about a specific client or client group;
- Child and Youth Workers participating in a community capacity building process.

Each of these scenarios presents its own set of professional issues. One reason why community involvement in child and youth care practice frequently is less substantial than it could be, and sometimes is barely present, is that practitioners often take an instrumental view of their engagement with the community. Such an approach creates limitations in terms of how we think about community and its role in child and youth care practice. It is therefore critical to explore some of the professional issues embedded in our work with community in some detail in order to ensure that our thinking about community presents us with as much opportunity as possible.

Child and youth workers often spend more time thinking about what the community has to offer to them and their clients than contemplating their relationship with the community. And yet we find that there are quite a number of questions that can be explored that are, in essence, relational questions. One of the issues in developing a child and youth worker approach to community engagement is how the child and youth worker sees himself or herself in relation to the community and how the community might perceive the presence of the child and youth worker. The first set of questions in need of some contemplation therefore is this:

- Am I part of the community or am I a visitor/guest/intruder?
- Am I a consumer of services in this community or am I a provider of services?
- What is my *responsibility* to the community?
- What is the community's responsibility towards me?

- What is my *accountability* to the community?
- What is the community's accountability towards me?

There is a significant difference between engaging the community in which one lives versus engaging a community where one has professional interests. In the former case, our professional activities with respect to community engagement transcend our professional role and impact us professionally and personally, whereas in the latter case we can maintain a degree of separation between the personal and the professional. From the perspective of the practitioner, this makes a difference in terms of how we might define the parameters of community engagement; we are, after all, engaging ourselves as members of the community if it is the community where we live. From the perspective of the community, it can add credibility to our advocacy on behalf of clients if indeed we are advocating within our own life spaces. It can also result in challenges associated with blending professional activities and obligations with personal relationships with neighbors, the staff at the community recreation center we use ourselves, or the political representatives of the community.

If, for example, we want to introduce a client with a history of sexual offending into the community through admission to our program, our advocacy on behalf of the client might well be tempered by our considerations for the safety of our own children if this happens to be the community where we live. When introducing such a client into a community where we work, on the other hand, the force of our advocacy often seems so much less inhibited. In the absence of an impact on our personal life space, we can advocate on behalf of this client within the protective field of the "moral high ground."

In the case of a noncontiguous community, such as a particular ethnic group, our advocacy for clients also is impacted by whether or not we self-identify as members of this community. Introducing a client into the ethnic community to which we ourselves belong presents quite different issues and challenges than introducing a client into a "stranger community" to which the client might belong but one that is strange to us. From our perspective, the criteria for community acceptance for this client ought to be his or her ethnic identity. From the community's perspective, a range of other factors might also be relevant, but we might struggle recognizing the legitimacy of such factors given that we are on the outside of this particular community. In cases such as this, it is critically important to be conscious of how the community might perceive us. Are we simply nonmembers, or could we even be seen as intruders or unwelcome guests? Are there historical or broader social barriers we might have to take into account? Examples that quickly come to mind might include issues of racism, religious animosity, and socioeconomic disparities.

These kinds of questions then lead to further questions related to responsibility and accountability. Our very presence in the community, professionally or personally, results in assuming some level of responsibility to the community. If we are to hold responsibility within the community, can we expect the community to hold responsibility toward us? And what will be the system of accountability by which these forms of responsibility are implemented, monitored and evaluated?

If we focus our contemplations more specifically on issues related to diversity and issues of oppression, we might further ask the following questions:

• Am I culturally competent to engage with this community?
• Do I present a threat to this community as a result of identity differences?
• How am I impacting on pre-existing tension related to diversity issues in this community?

Further, recognizing that our presence as practitioners always entails an impact of the balance of power, whether in relation of a child, a family, or the community, we might contemplate the following kinds of questions as well:

• Am I a source of empowerment in this community?
• Am I a source of disempowerment in this community?
• Am I feeling empowered or disempowered by this community?
• Do I understand how power functions in this community?

In thinking about these questions, we are mirroring the process that takes place when we develop relationships either with children or with families (Molepo, 2005). Community relationships tend to take on more of the complexities of relationships with families in part because communities are never entirely uniform or undifferentiated. There is diversity within all communities, sometimes visible and sometimes less so. Our interactions with and engagement of that diversity, therefore, has to take account of the resources and needs of each center of identity and social group within the community. Far from being an instrumental issue, a child and youth care approach to community engagement is therefore a relational approach that begins with considerable contemplation about where and how our relationship with the community is positioned. In so doing, we can identify a range of very practical issues that need to be considered both before we begin our engagement with the community and throughout the life of that engagement. Much like working with a family, we have to be conscious of issues such as boundaries, confidentiality and communication (Barter, 2003; Martin & Tennant, 2008; Rauner, 2000).

Boundaries

While we are engaging with the community in relation to a particular client or family, we may well encounter demands on our services from members of the community in relation to their specific concerns and needs; how do we define our limits? Alternatively, there might be services in the community that we use ourselves but that we can readily identify as potentially useful for our clients; to what degree do we allow our personal life to become exposed to the client by sharing community services with the client? When we connect a client to a community to which we ourselves belong, such as the gay community, how will we respond when the client participates in some of the same festivities or community events we do? What will happen when the client gains access to some of the same people we know? While we can control our approach to confidentiality, will those people talk about us to the client?

Confidentiality

In order to ensure that specific community services or programs do not have preconceived notions about our clients or us, we may have to disclose information in order to provide a better understanding of the circumstances that have led us to connect with the client in the first place. This will raise myriad issues in relation to confidentiality. In some cases, we might be able to work with the client in delineating the extent of information we are allowed to disclose. In other cases, however, clients may lack the capacity to provide such input and we will have to make decisions about disclosure based on ethical principles, policies and procedures and our more pragmatic interest in getting the client access to services. In these cases, we have to weigh the benefits of access against the potential drawbacks of having services be delivered with the client's uniqueness and its implications interpreted by a range of individuals in different ways.

Confidentiality in the context of community engagement can take myriad other forms as well. Particularly if we are engaging the community where we ourselves live, the odds of coming into contact with personal connections while with the clients are increased significantly. How do we introduce the client to our friends? To what degree do we want the client to gain access to or even to be aware of our personal connections in the community? Another scenario that might unfold relates to crises with the client in the community. What if we have to physically contain the client and onlookers rush to her side to assist? How much information can we provide in order to diffuse such a situation and to protect ourselves against possible violent interventions on the part of community members?

Communication

All communities feature a range of approaches to communicating ideas and articulating values. While there may well be community values that can be generalized and applied to the patterns of interaction and social functioning of a larger social grouping, one typically also encounters articulations of counter-values and frequently anti-social, racist, homophobic, sexist, or otherwise oppressive and exclusionary ways toward individuals or minority groups within the community. The challenge for the child and youth worker will be how and when to respond to these situations. All communities have strengths and weaknesses and our clients will likely be exposed to both. As professionals operating within the community, therefore, we may well have a responsibility to respond to negative dynamics and provide positive alternatives to those initiating such dynamics. On the other hand, it is not always easy or even safe to respond to someone espousing negativity in the moment. And yet, our clients will look to us as role models, and they may well expect us to respond even when we are not entirely comfortable doing so.

It becomes clear, then, that community engagement within the day-to-day activities of child and youth care practitioners is complex and undertaken with much to consider. Far from being simply an instrumental component of the job, the very presence of community in our life spaces and in the life spaces of the child raises many challenges, opportunities, and dilemmas with respect to how and when we might engage the community. Much like our relationships with children and families, our relationship with the community is governed by dynamics related to boundaries, the exploration of Self and our understanding of the relational interconnectivities within the community we are engaging.

While the context of community engagement is very complex, the motivation for engaging communities is often much simpler and based on immediate needs. One of the most common reasons for child and youth workers to engage within the community relates to accessing services for clients or matching clients with the right services at the right time.

FINDING SERVICES FOR OUR CLIENTS

Whether they live in the community or in residential settings, isolation is a common challenge for the children and families with whom child and youth workers are engaged. The need to connect with community services and find ways of incorporating children and families into these services is great. This raises several professional issues that often are covered by job descriptions and the pronouncements of agency values and mission statements but that at the same time often are sidelined by the many moment-to-moment responsibilities of the practitioner. In seeking services for our clients, the first step for the practitioner is to be educated about the services that are available in the community. This is in and of itself a challenging task and not one that many child and youth care practitioners are prepared to do. In many communities there are no systematic guides to community services available, and, therefore much of the knowledge about specific services is spread through word of mouth. In such communities, the importance of being exposed to the community is greatly enhanced, since without such exposure, finding out about specific services becomes even more challenging. In other communities, there are in fact compilations of community services available, often in the form of on-line databases that can be accessed by everyone. Even in these communities, however, very few practitioners are aware of the full range of services at any given time. Instead, practitioners search for an appropriate service once the need for such service has been identified. While this is helpful, it does have the disadvantage that the use of community resources becomes limited to situations where specific needs have in fact been identified. The presence of community resources does not contribute to the early intervention in specific needs on the part of the child or the family.

It is common, for example, for a child to appear disengaged in his day-to-day activities and expectations within the family, at school, or within the context of a residential placement. An early intervention might provide the child with opportunities to participate in a wide range of community activities or programs in order to determine whether any might be of interest longer term. In the absence of being aware of community resources, child and youth care practitioners are not likely to encourage or assist with this process of exploration until the impact of the client's disengagement creates a need for intervention. At that point, particularly in those communities where the information is readily available, the practitioner might seek out an appropriate service as an intervention into an identified problem rather than as an early intervention to stave off a problem.

One of the professional issues for practitioners, therefore, relates to the ongoing responsibility to maintain knowledge and seek out new information about what is happening within the community. Practitioners must have knowledge of formal and institutionalized services as well as informal and grassroots services within the community in order to seek out services, programs, and resources on behalf of clients that maintain the focus on participation and engagement within the client's life spaces. One of the reasons why children and youth experience so much of their day-to-day activities in institutional and formal environments is that child and youth care practitioners are not sufficiently aware of what is happening in the community in a more informal, and therefore less marketed or advertised, format.

Seeking out community services on behalf of clients is not the same as assisting clients with gaining access to such services. Within the context of access, a number of major barriers can be encountered, including but not limited to the following:

• Cost of admission and access to equipment
• Stereotyping of client situations
• Racial and other stereotypes

- Client behaviors
- Safety considerations

Economic resources often present major barriers to creating access for children and youth to participate in specific activities. Especially in the context of recreational activities, the cost of registration and equipment can be substantial and ongoing, given that children typically outgrow their equipment quickly. For the child and youth care practitioner, seeking access to a particular service or program within the community, therefore, often requires accessing various other types of community resources in order to provide a foundation for ongoing access to the service or program sought out in the first place.

Additional challenges relate to stereotyping of client situations or even of client identity characteristics. For the practitioner, many of the professional issues discussed earlier pursuant to boundaries, confidentiality and communication within the context of community engagement therefore become activated. Preparedness to respond to such stereotyping is one of the core requirements for the practitioner. And, finally, notwithstanding the needs and the rights of all children to gain access to community-based services and programs, there often are behavioral issues and safety considerations that render such access legitimately challenging. We can, for example, imagine the impact of an extremely aggressive child entering a boys group; the group dynamics might be at risk and the experience of the other boys in the group might become seriously impaired. Again, the practitioner has a responsibility to coordinate community services from multiple sources in order to provide the support and resources required to ensure that the boy joining the group does not negate the purpose or function of the group. At the same time, the prejudice against children who have challenging behaviors cannot be a cause for exclusion, and the practitioner maintains responsibility for advocating on behalf of protecting the child from further disadvantage based on myths or presumptive judgment on the part of the service provider or community group.

In some cases, negotiating access for children can also raise ethical dilemmas for the practitioner. In referring a sexual offender to a community program where there are potentially vulnerable children, the practitioner has to weigh the rights of the client to have access to the community against the rights of the other children to be safe.

Blind advocacy on behalf of one's client is not a virtuous activity if it places other children at significant risk of harm.

RESPONDING TO COMMUNITY CONCERNS

Another way in which child and youth care practitioners frequently engage with the community relates to responding to community concerns. Particularly in a residential context, neighbors and community members often are adversely impacted by the actions of the children or youth residing in the program. Whether the residents are yelling profanities in the neighborhood, smoking in front of the house or engaging in unsightly activities, neighbors are frequently quick to complain. In these situations, child and youth care practitioners often try to diffuse conflict by either denying the residents' responsibility or more commonly, by "consequencing" the residents for their actions. This can even entail consequences that restrict community access for the residents so as to avoid further conflict for the time being.

In addition to the actions on the part of the residents that directly impact the neighborhood, sometimes it is the actions of residents that result in a frequent police or ambulance presence at the residential program that cause alarm in the neighborhood and results in complaints or at least inquiries about what is happening in the group home. As a result of confidentiality issues, child and youth workers often are limited in what they feel they can disclose to the neighbors, resulting in a neighborhood feeling of mistrust and suspicion.

Clearly these reactive approaches to dealing with community concerns are not particularly useful or effective. When programs find themselves subject to repeated complaints or even neighborhood movements to have the program closed or relocated, it often reflects a lack of relational engagement between the child and youth workers and the neighbors. In fact, many of the ongoing neighborhood issues can much more effectively be dealt with when practitioners recognize the importance of community engagement as an integral part of their job. Conflict is much more easily resolved in the context of an ongoing relationship governed by at least some degree of transparency and trust than when all interactions between the parties to the conflict unfold in the context of problems. The professional issues that are embedded within this specific context of community engagement, then, once again relate to the professional requirement for practitioners to actively seek out relational engagement with the community. The challenge associated with this is that often there is little agency support for practitioners doing so on an ongoing basis. A lack of support might be related to an agency's history of operating in isolation from the community but more often is related to a lack of resources for child and youth workers to have the time to introduce themselves and interact with the neighbors and other members of the community outside of their shift schedule.

A proactive, relational engagement with key community stakeholders is not only a core component of residential work. Even practitioners who work with families in their homes, or those who work with children and youth in recreation centers or in the community, would benefit a great deal from making connections with some of the core stakeholders such as police officers, local businesses and other social service providers. An understanding that quality child and youth care practice requires the practitioner to engage and be engaged with the community and specific stakeholders within that community thus constitutes a core component of professional practice.

A NEW ROLE FOR CHILD AND YOUTH CARE PRACTITIONERS

So far, we have explored primarily the *reactive* approach to community engagement, based either on having identified specific needs of clients and therefore seeking out appropriate services, or responding to community complaints or concerns. It is also possible to think about community engagement in more *proactive* ways. In so doing, practitioners may find ways of not only being relationally engaged with community but also of enhancing what is possible within community; in other words, when we begin to think about community engagement in proactive terms, it becomes a field of opportunity rather than a dreaded obligation. One increasingly common framework for engaging community in a proactive way is referred to as community capacity building (CCB). CCB has traditionally been perceived as a professional function of the social work discipline supported in part by the community development stream of graduate social work schools. Child and youth workers, in contrast, speak of community-based work, which, as we discussed earlier, typically means engaging in direct service activities with children, youth or families outside of institutional settings.

The fundamental premises of CCB mirror at least some of the core principles of child and youth care practice. CCB is based on the belief that all communities, no matter how marginalized, have strengths or assets that could give rise to healthy and functional day-to-day experiences within the community. This certainly mirrors the strengths-based approach and focus on resilience typical of child and youth care practice. In addition, CCB seeks to engender social processes that unfold and impact locally on those involved in the process; again, a close resemblance to the child and youth care concept of "the centrality of life spaces": "Capacity building refers to the means by which a community can tap into its own strengths... It is not possible for 'outsiders' to come into a community and create capacity. Capacity building is not likely unless the community has the assets to begin with and the will to mobilize these assets" (Austin, 2004, n.p.).

Not all articulations of CCB mirror the core concepts of child and youth care practice. In some versions, CCB is indeed seen as a process developed for a community from the outside of that community. In fact, this is sometimes seen as the major difference between what has long been referred to as community development (CD) and CCB (Atkinson & Willis, 2006). Fundamentally, however, the framework of CCB allows for child and youth care practitioners to explore their relationship with the community in ways that transcend the instrumentality of seeking services or responding to community concerns, and instead to enhance their relational engagement with the community. The rationale for incorporating community capacity building functions into the professional portfolio of child and youth care is substantial, and it finds justification in the vast majority of community needs assessments and community gap analyses conducted across North America and beyond.

In recent years, multiple studies (Hastings, 2001; Hanvey et al., 1994; McMurty & Curling, 2008) have demonstrated that in both urban and rural settings throughout North America one of the greatest gaps in community capacity pertains specifically to living with youth. Both within the family unit and within institutional settings such as schools and social service organizations (children's mental health and child welfare), youth are presenting challenges that often cannot be addressed effectively from within the particular setting in which such challenges emerge; although a community response is clearly needed, none is typically available. Gap analyses in many communities across North America point clearly and repetitiously to the absence or inadequacies of many or even all of the following:

- Early intervention services, crisis supports and ongoing and intensive support for chronic needs
- Alternative to custody programs and accountability measures
- Residential and nonresidential respite opportunities
- Educational supports and assessment and early identification of Learning Disabilities
- Addiction services and counseling services (that are accessible)
- Social infrastructure including recreation centers, affordable housing, income supports, and the like
- Culturally competent social services

Given the focus on youth within the evolution, development, and implementation of community capacity building initiatives, there is increasing justification for the deployment of *child and youth workers as capacity builders* rather than only as *service providers* within a capacity-building program that may or may not be compatible with the child and youth work approaches commonly applied in community-based child and youth work. As indicated, the process of community capacity building includes significant overlap with some of the fundamental principles of relational child and youth work. For one thing, this process shares the belief that change, strength, and resilience are built from within the community (the family or the child) but always in the context of the community's physical, social, and cultural characteristics (in the life spaces of the child or family). In fact, much like a systems view of family functioning, community capacity building presumes that the *process* of community functioning and its physical, social, and cultural *contexts* are interdependent.

We also discussed a little earlier that community engagement requires an awareness of one's own role within the community, not only in an instrumental way, but also in terms of the meaning and implication of our presence within the community. CCB, in turn, incorporates the presence of the capacity builders as an active component of the process rather than an external factor impacting on the community independently from its role within the community. In this sense, the child and youth worker engaged with the community in a capacity building process, much like the child and youth worker engaged with a family, becomes connected to the social, physical and cultural spaces of that community through her or his own presence alone.

THREE ACCESS POINTS TO PROACTIVE COMMUNITY WORK

In the introduction to this article, community was presented as an important yet profoundly underutilized resource in child and youth care practice. One reason why child and youth care practitioners appear at best moderately engaged with the communities of the children, youth and families they work with is their uncertainty about how to access these communities. As a way of facilitating the transition of community as a concept to community as an active element of one's practice, we can identify at least three access points to communities that are readily available to the practitioner: the peer group, neighbors, and the police.

Peer Groups

Every child, youth, and family has peer groups, and in the vast majority of situations, the peer group is present within the home community of the child or youth. It would seem obvious that being present within the peer context of our clients constitutes a major element of engaging in life space practice. Indeed, peer group engagement provides opportunities to be present in the community through activity-based approaches to impacting on peer group dynamics and facilitating positive peer to peer relationships. Given that very often behavioral challenges associated with our client are based on peer influences and sometimes poor group decision-making amongst the peers, child and youth care practitioners have a vested interest in gaining access to this critical life space of the child or youth. In addition, engagement with peer groups also provides opportunities for engagement with the peers' families; in this way, the practitioner becomes entrenched in community life through the medium that is most familiar to him—relationships.

Neighbors

Every child, youth, and family has neighbors, whether they live in detached homes or in apartment complexes. For many families, neighborly relations are strained, sometimes because of the stigma attached to having involvements with social services or the helping professions. Often, there is also an embarrassment factor for families who are not particularly proud of having to seek the assistance of professionals to deal with family conflict or parenting challenges. Ethno-racial, cultural, and language factors might also be relevant in many situations. The practitioner, therefore, has to remain sensitive of the family's perception of the neighborhood and neighborly relations; however, this does not mean that an engagement with neighbors should be ruled out from the start. In practice, almost everybody has some level of engagement with their neighbors. Given the constant presence of neighbors in the lives of our clients, it makes sense to be concerned about how this presence is impacting on our clients. Even silent conflict can become a stressor in the day-to-day functioning of families and the experiences of children and youth. Once again, therefore, the practitioner has an opportunity to use his relational skills in engaging with the neighbors. Everyday acknowledgments of the neighbors' presence, introductions by first name, and participation in neighborhood events all serve to facilitate developing neighborly relationships that are inclusive, transparent and meaningful for everyone concerned.

Police and Security Personnel

Police involvement either directly with our clients or indirectly through a presence in the neighborhood is a fact of life for many of our clients. For families living in public housing clusters or in large apartment complexes, security personnel may also be visibly present most of the time. Most of the time, child and youth care practitioners engage with police or security personnel in a reactive manner, after an incident or during an investigation. Yet police and security personnel can also be engaged proactively and, in many cases, can be motivated to serve as positive relationships for the children and youth with whom we work. The stress associated with interacting with these professionals reactively can be mitigated by establishing prior relationships. Once again, personal introductions, day-to-day acknowledgments of their presence, and invitations to participate in activities or events are simple things that a child and youth care practitioner can do in order to gain access to this very important element in the life space of the client.

Incorporating a strong consciousness of community in the day-to-day activities of child and youth care practitioners creates opportunities for enriching the child and youth care experience. While a relational engagement with community gives rise to many professional issues for the practitioner, there is no question that the opportunities that will present themselves through the engagement of community render it worthwhile to seek resolution of such professional issues. Particularly in the context of the proactive CCB approach, child and youth care practitioners can substantially enhance the impact of their profession, which would benefit the practitioners as much as the children, youth and families who rely on them for assistance, motivation and hope.

REFERENCES

Atkinson, R., & Willis, P. (2006). *Community capacity building: A practical guide.* Retrieved May 31, 2009, from www.utas.edu.au/sociology/HACRU/6%20 Community%20Capacity%20building.pdf

Austin, P. (2004). *Community capacity building and mobilization in youth mental health promotion.* Retrieved January 31, 2009, from http://www.phac-aspc.gc.ca/mh-sm/mhp-psm/pub/community-communautaires/index-eng.php#2

Banks, S. (1993). Community youth work. In H. Butcher, A. Glen, P. Henderson, & J. Smith (Eds.), *Community and public policy* (pp. 71–87). London: Pluto Press.

Barter, K. (2003). Strengthening community capacity: Expanding the vision. *Relational Child and Youth Care Practice, 16*(2), 24–32.

Hastings, R. (2001). *Community mobilization and crime prevention.* Draft Report to the National Crime Prevention Centre. Ottawa, Canada: Department of Justice.

Hanvey, L. H., Avard, D., Graham, I., Underwood, K., Campbell, J., & Kelly, C. (1994). *The health of Canada's children: A CICH profile* (2nd ed.). Ottawa, Canada: Canadian Institute of Child Health.

Kover Kline, K. (Ed.) (2008). *Authoritative communities: The scientific case for nurturing the whole child.* New York: Springer.

Mannes, M., Roehlkepartain, E., & Benson, P. (2005). Unleashing the power of community to strengthen the well being of children, youth and families: An asset building approach. *Child Welfare, 84*(2), 233–250.

Martin, D., & Tennant, G. (2008). Child and youth care in the community center. *Relational Child and Youth Care Practice, 21*(2), 20–26

McElwee, N. (2007). *At risk children & youth: Resiliency explored.* New York: Haworth Press.

McKnight, J. (1995). *The careless society: Community and its counterfeits.* New York: Basic Books.

McMurty, R., & Curling, A. (2008). *Roots of youth violence.* Toronto, Canada: Service Ontario Publications.

Molepo, L. (2005). Community child and youth care work: The unspecified therapeutic aspects. *Relational Child and Youth Care Practice, 18*(2) 14–17.

Pittman, K. (2000). Balancing the equation: Communities supporting youth, youth supporting communities. *Community Youth Development Journal, 133–36.*

Rauner, D. M. (2000). *The role of caring in youth development and community life.* New York: Columbia University Press.

Scales, P. C., Benson, P. L., Roehlkepartain, E. C., Hintz, N. R., Sullivan, T. K. et al. (2001). The role of neighborhood and community in building developmental assets for children and youth: A national study of social norms among American adults. *Journal of Community Psychology, 29,* 703–727.

Smale, G. G. (1995). Integrating community and individual practice: A new paradigm for practice. In P. Adams & K. Nelson (Eds.), *Reinventing human services: Community-and family-centered practice* (pp. 59–80). New York: Aldine De Gruyter.

Ungar, M. (Ed.). (2004). *Handbook for working with children and youth: Pathways to resilience across cultures and contexts.* London: SAGE.

Professional Issues of Child and Youth Care Through the Language Lens

SUMMARY. This article explores the role of language and forms of communication in professional child and youth care practice. It is argued that all the professional issues of child and youth care practice are significantly impacted by language and the manner in which practitioners use language and a variety of communication forms to articulate their work. The role of jargon in child and youth care practice is examined using several commonly used terms as examples. The need for an ongoing, critical perspective in the use of language is emphasized, and practitioners are encouraged to contemplate the biases and unexamined truths embedded in their day-to-day language use.

KEYWORDS. Biases, child and youth work, communication, jargon, language, professional issues, truth, voice

Child and youth care practitioners spend a great deal of their time "talking"; they talk to their clients, to members of the community, to each other and to other professionals. Any exploration of the major professional issues in child and youth care practice exposes the centrality of language in the profession. The profession is socially engaged and interaction with others is necessary in order for the practitioner to fulfill his duties. As Batsleer (2008, p. 8) points out,

"Since language is the main vehicle of conversation, committed practitioners need to have a keen awareness of language and talk, its different registers and tones and the nature of communication in talk." There are many obvious connections between language and professional issues. For example, practitioners generally know that the use of profanity while having discussions with other professionals is not desirable. They also know that different levels of language formality are required depending on the audience. During team discussions involving a close group of child and youth care practitioners, it may be possible to use colloquial language, casual expressions, and language that presumes familiarity with professional jargon. In the context of a multi-disciplinary case conference, on the other hand, the level of language must be higher, jargon must be avoided, and articulating one's point of view must reflect language usage that is commensurate with the standards set by other professionals.

In addition to these obvious professional issues related to language, there are many that are either less obvious or that have been complacently accepted as non-issues. It is in this context that the profession of child and youth care practice is exposed to an ongoing risk of being labeled a "second tier" or a "quasi-profession" by other professionals, by community stakeholders and perhaps even by families and youth. As practitioners, it is worthwhile to contemplate our use of language, collectively and individually, in order to ensure that we are representing our work as we think we are; it is, after all, a common wisdom that "what is said is not necessarily what is heard." In this article, therefore, we will explore some of the biases and jargons that are often contained in our language use, and we will consider the implications of engaging in an uncritical use of language. Finally, we will explore some of the strategies that can help mitigate the language dilemmas we frequently face in our practice.

CHILD AND YOUTH CARE JARGON

While professionals in all disciplines, and certainly including child and youth care practitioners, pay a great deal of attention to their forms of communication, much less attention is paid to the language that provides the substance for the communication process. It is no exaggeration to suggest that as a field, we have often taken language for granted. Perhaps this is the result of the field being relatively new and therefore having borrowed its language for many decades from other fields, including psychology, sociology and social work. It really has only been in the past fifty years or so that the field of child and youth care has developed its own language, prompting some to advocate for the development of a shared language between the professions and the families they serve (Casson, 2005).

Language is not value neutral (Samovar, Porter, & McDaniel, 2007). Quite to the contrary, virtually all the power imbalances within our society are embedded within language. While we can express many positive things through the use of language, we also have to recognize that the core tool used in all negative dynamics within our society are accompanied by a language specifically designed to perpetuate negativity (Perry, 2006; Sayer, 2008; Suderman, 2007). Racism, sexism, homophobia and oppression more generally all are anchored by language that expresses biases as truths, inequalities as norms, and virtue as reflective of one or another dominant perspective (DeGenaro, 2007).

Many of the expressions we use in child and youth care also reflect unexamined ideas about truths. We can consider, for example, terms such as "struggle," "success," "appropriate" or even "good." A critical contemplation of common uses of these terms in practice settings quickly establishes some of the unexamined truths and assumptions generated by this language. When we identify a child or youth as struggling, what are we really identifying? How do we know it is the child struggling and not the worker or the program struggling? In the context of a classic power struggle between a child and a child and youth worker, who really has the problem? Is it the vulnerable child who has relatively little power to choose, few options for action and many constraints that are imposed by program expectations, legal parameters and often physical force? Or is it the child and youth worker, who has professional training, gets paid to be there, can look forward to some downtime after the end of her shift and, at any time, can choose to take a vacation in sun-filled Mexico to recover from the stress at work? In contemplating these questions, it is important to recognize that this is not a trivial issue but, instead, it is an issue that drives our thinking about much more fundamental concepts such as strength-based approaches to practice, resilience, and even diagnostic considerations. Equating noncompliance with "struggle" on the part of the child negates possibilities that we take for granted in our own lives. For example, it is not uncommon for us to be noncompliant in many of our life spaces. Many of us might have broken traffic rules by exceeding the speed limit or coming to a rolling stop at a stop sign. We typically break rules as a result of a cost–benefit analysis and what we might consider a reasonable assessment of risk. If we speed, we will get to our destination more quickly and the chance of getting a speeding ticket is low; therefore we proceed with breaking the rule that we are fully aware of. We would not typically associate this kind of decision-making with the concept of "struggle." And yet, when a child or youth breaks the rules in the context of a residential program or a classroom setting, we are quick to label the child or youth as "struggling" with respect to the expectations of the program, thus negating the possibility that the child or youth is making reasonable assessments of the risks and engaged in a sophisticated cost–benefit analysis.

While the focus on compliance in many child and youth care practice contexts is not entirely a function of language, but also includes (often without evidence) assumptions about clinical values and outcomes, articulating the absence of compliance as "struggle" has serious implications in how we do our work and how that work will impact on the client. Compliance is not always a good thing; excessive compliance can raise the risk of abuse and other negative outcomes (Fox, 1994). Compliance can also mitigate coping strategies that children and youth adopt in order to live with and overcome adversity. Chronic running, for example, has increasingly been recognized as potentially symptomatic not of behavior problems but of coping strategies. We therefore distinguish now between "running from" something and "running to" something as a way of providing at least for the possibility that running away might be an indication of strength. In many practice settings, the view that running away is inherently a problematic behavior diminishes the value of decision-making and resilience of the client and negates the possibility that it is the program that is struggling to provide a meaningful service rather than the client struggling with remaining present in a service that is unhelpful and potentially even harmful.

When it comes to identifying "success," what criteria are we using? Are we talking about success through the eyes of the child or youth, or are we measuring success based on criteria deemed important by us or by some articulation of societal norms? Is success really just a matter of clients acting within the expected parameters of whatever program they are enrolled in? Who gets to determine what constitutes success? While outcome studies of services apply a more complex and sophisticated program evaluation approach to delineating success, at the level of the practitioner success is frequently equated with "doing well" in the program. As such, the individuality of clients and their unique ways of experiencing success is diminished, and instead we adopt a more programmatic and "objective" assessment. Conversely, when clients are not doing well in the program, we are quick to label this as "failure," in part because the commitment to helping clients achieving success requires the acceptance of its opposite. Much like imposing the term "struggle" on clients based on our criteria, the use of the term "success" is profoundly disempowering to the client and therefore has much wider implications then simply creating an issue of semantics. When practitioners adopt the language of success and failure based on pre-determined sets of criteria (often perform-ance-related criteria), the very concept of client empowerment is essentially negated.

We can similarly point out that the designation of "appropriate" is an entirely relative designation. Nothing is inherently appropriate; things can only be appropriate in relation to a pre-determined set of norms. Why is it inappropriate for a 17-year-old youth living in a group home to swear in their common language, but there is really not a problem when a group of 18-year-old university students use extensive profanity in their informal chatter? And even the term "good" reflects biases and unexamined correlations to terms such as "success." If a child is "good," success will follow. Conversely, success implies "goodness." But does it really? Is "being good" a descriptor of behaviors or a moral assessment? Does it reflect the child's happiness or the child and youth worker's measure of control and power resulting from the child's compliance? Can success in selling drugs be described as "good?" If not, why not? Such success does, after all, reflect a high level of performance in a complex task.

DECONSTRUCTING THE LANGUAGE OF CORE CONCEPTS

Jargon exists in abundance in most professional disciplines. Given the centrality of language and communication in the child and youth care discipline, however, the importance of remaining conscious of jargon and its implications is greatly elevated. For practitioners, the issue is not simply one of potentially being misunderstood by others; it is also an issue of misrepresenting the identity, capacities and possibilities of children and youth in their relationships to adults and to their life spaces. Practitioners therefore have a responsibility to mitigate the impact of jargon within the discipline and to remain critically engaged with their language use. What becomes readily apparent is that virtually everything we say is embedded in the many assumptions and biases of language. We use our value-laden language not only to communicate with one another or with the children and youth we serve but also to draw conclusions about what we have accomplished and how we might proceed. As soon as we express a thought through language, we have done several things, including the following:

- Invited a response from others;
- Created an agenda for ourselves and others;
- Labeled someone or something;
- Excluded a million other possibilities in describing someone or something;
- Committed ourselves to a particular way of seeing the world, at least at that particular moment;
- Relinquished control over our thought because while we have some control over what we say we have very little control over what is heard.

Mitigating the impact of language on the practice of child and youth workers requires more than an identification of jargon terms. It requires that core concepts of the discipline are re-examined with a view of establishing the potential contradictions and dilemmas embedded within these concepts. It is only when we take a conceptual approach to our work that critically examines our practices through a variety of lenses that we can begin to take action in order to mitigate some of the imperfections necessarily entailed in a profession based so fundamentally on communication. By way of example, we will examine three core concepts of the profession in some detail. The goal is to take these concepts and "de-construct" some of the unexamined truths often assumed about these concepts. Specifically, we will explore the concepts of "caring," "relationship," and "engagement" through the language lens.

Caring

The term "caring" has been at the core of our profession in rather obvious ways forever. If we just think about the various professional titles for our discipline, the word "care" appears to be quite prevalent. Ryerson University in Toronto refers to its program as the School of Child and Youth Care Practice; one of the leading journals in the field is called *Relational Child and Youth Care Practice*; another journal is called the *Journal of Child and Youth Care Work*; and many employers refer to us as Child Care Workers, Child and Youth Care Workers or even Direct Care Workers. But what does it really mean when we speak of "caring" in child and youth care practice?

The language of caring really covers two entirely different things. On the one hand, it is a reference to caring *about someone*, while on the other hand, it is also a reference to caring *for someone*. Caring about someone has a significant emotional connotation, and linguistically, terms such as empathy, pity, feelings, and love come to mind. The idea of caring for someone, in contrast, is very much an action oriented idea, and linguistically, we might think of terms such as caretaking, providing for basic needs, and health care. Caring about someone is hardly considered a professional activity. Sure, many professionals in the social and human services presumably care about their clients, but so do nice people everywhere: philanthropists, the rich and famous, and anyone who has a big heart and is somewhat socially conscious. Caring for someone is certainly considered an activity, but whether or not it is a professional one depends on who is doing it. On one end of the spectrum is high end medical care, and doctors, nurses, psychiatrists, and perhaps others might well be considered to be engaging in a professional activity when providing care within the boundaries of their discipline. But many other people also provide care for others, including adults for their aging parents, parents for their children, and home care workers for the elderly or those with physical disabilities.

So what exactly does it mean when child and youth care workers talk about "caring for kids?" In some cases, we might be able to translate this idea quite literally. Given that more and more child and youth workers are employed in settings where self care is an issue for clients (such as Acquired Brain Injury programs, programs for individuals with autism, and myriad programs traditionally considered to be Disability Services programs), physically caring for children and youth may well be one of the job requirements for these child and youth workers. On the other hand, the majority of child and youth workers still work in settings where these activities are not typically part of the daily tasks, including classrooms, group homes, recreation centers, custody settings, and shelters for homeless youth. What does caring for someone mean in those settings?

Perhaps it means caring for the emotional needs of the child or youth, or perhaps it means caring for their educational needs, or their health and nutrition needs, or their mental health needs, or any other sort of needs. But how do we do that? What actions are involved in doing so, and how do we know whether these actions in fact have the effect of the child or youth being cared for? Is caring for a child simply a shorter way of saying that we get the kids through their daily routines and manage the expectations of whatever program we are working in? Or is the provision of care at the hands of a child and youth worker an inherent by-product of the institutional care provided by larger sectors? In the child welfare system in North America, for example, children are said to be either "in care" or "out of care." Surely this does not mean that if children are out of care they are not being cared for.

How do child and youth workers care for children and youth? When a child needs health care, we take him or her to the doctor. When educational care is needed, we send her or him to school. When the needs are emotional, we make an appointment with the counsellor. For mental health care, off to the psychiatrist we go. So other than transporting the child to various places where care can be received, what do we do? Of course, ensuring that a child gets the appropriate care from the appropriate professional at the appropriate time is in and of itself a way of caring for someone. But is this considered to be a professional activity? Is this not what parents do for their children every single day?

We can think about the relationship between caring for and caring about the child or youth differently. As mentioned previously, we generally assume that we care about the children and youth we work with. It is therefore noteworthy that Gerry Fewster (2005) once wrote an editorial titled "I don't like kids." His point was simply that the work we do should not be contingent on whether or not we like a child. For all kinds of perfectly normal and healthy reasons, some children will appeal to us more than others, but we have to provide the highest standard of practice for each and every child we encounter regardless of this. "Liking" is not the same as caring about someone, but it is pretty close. So, is it possible to care for someone about whom we do not care? Conversely, is it possible to care about someone but be ineffective in caring for that person? The answer to both these questions is probably a resounding YES! That means that when we say something like "child and youth work is fundamentally about caring," we are saying virtually nothing at all, and instead, we might be raising far more questions than we are answering.

After playing some language games with the concept of caring it turns out that the intuitive understanding of this term may not capture a great deal of content when it comes to child and youth work. Somehow, if we are to ensure that there is a common and meaningful understanding of this core concept amongst ourselves and other professionals, we will have to reflect on its meaning in somewhat more complex ways. Our greatest fear is and ought to be that we have come to *think* about this concept in as unproblematic way as we *articulate* it.

Relationships

Not too long ago in our history as a field of practice, a child and youth worker might have responded to the question about what he does as follows: *I hang out with kids who have problems, I try to teach them right from wrong, but mostly I try to make sure they have fun while they're waiting to see what's next in their lives.*

Today, this type of response is probably not good enough. A number of major changes have taken hold over the course of the past two decades:

- We cannot just "hang out with kids and try to have fun"; what we do is prescribed by management and multidisciplinary team expectations, as well as by policies and procedures, by the expectations of monitored Plans of Care, and by the resolutions of case conferences.
- Our role is much less isolated than it used to be and our reporting of what kids are up to on a day-to-day basis is used in decision-making in the context of family court, criminal court, schools, probation, community services, and even assessments.

- Our own demands for recognition as professionals with specific skills and a repertoire of interventions has resulted in the need to justify our role in a language that corresponds in quality and vocabulary to the language of other professionals.

In response to some of these changes, we have adopted the term "relationship" as a way of thinking about our involvement with children and youth and therefore also articulating that involvement to others. Given the ever-rising profile of issues such as boundaries and confidentiality, we have modified the term by adding the prefix "therapeutic." So what used to be described as "hanging out with kids" is now referred to as developing therapeutic relationships with children, youth and sometimes families.

One of the immediate challenges arising from this use of language is that the term "relationship" refers to a state of *being* in relation to someone else but not to any particular activity with respect to that someone else. For others outside of the child and youth care profession, the question arises as to why we should get paid to just "be" with the child; specifically, what skills are involved in "being?" Couldn't the same value be had by recruiting volunteers to do this?

Perhaps the secret is to focus on the term "therapeutic" more so than on the term "relationship." What does therapeutic mean? What are we thinking about when we use this term? How do we convey those thoughts to others? Perhaps therapeutic means to have a relationship that promotes healing and growth. Or maybe it means that the relationship is part of therapy. Perhaps a therapeutic relationship is one that promotes change in the social systems around the child. Maybe it promotes change in the way the child views her surrounding systems and interacts with them. Or is it perhaps also possible that the relationship is therapeutic for us rather than the child, in the sense that it simply makes us feel better about the challenges faced by the child? What are we thinking about when we try to articulate what we do using the term "relationship?" What is the purpose of relationships? And how do we turn that purpose into meaningful child and youth care practice?

One way of thinking about the purpose of developing relationships with children and youth is to facilitate a double process: On the one hand, a process by which the child increases her ability to receive something (caring, nurturance, support, guidance); and on the other hand, the process of the child and youth worker giving something (his presence, affection, wisdom, comfort). Recognizing this double process in our thinking is an important first step in finding ways to articulate what we do in terms of relationships. A number of possibilities present themselves:

- Although "relationships" are about *being* in relation to someone, the processes of giving and receiving are in fact actions and, like all actions, the carrying out of these requires some level of understanding and skill.
- Child and youth care practice is somewhat unique in its dual focus on the child's ability to receive and the worker's ability to give. It is based on a recognition that in the absence of either one of these, not much change can happen from a developmental perspective.
- Relationships are another way of denoting *connections*, and the more open a connection the more information can flow through it. In this sense, our use of relationships is based on a desire to maximize the child's opportunity for learning and growth through the acquisition of new ways of seeing things.

If we think about some of these possibilities, we can consider the meaning of commonly used phrases in child and youth care practice somewhat differently. For example, many child and youth workers have been heard saying something like this:

I have a good relationship with little Eric.
Eric has trouble forming relationships.
I spent some one-on-one time with Eric to build a relationship with him.

The first phrase seems fine enough, describing what the worker believes to be the nature of his relationship with a child. Yet, it is interesting in and of itself to think for a moment about whether or not relationships can in fact be "good" or "bad." Or is it possible that relationships are value-neutral but how a child or a worker is experiencing that relationship is positive or negative or easy or challenging? This invokes a common scenario in child and youth worker team settings, where one worker tends to be fairly *laissez faire* while others are consistent and firm with the rules and program expectations. A common view of this situation is that the *laissez faire* worker is developing his relationship with the child by sabotaging the other workers. The child obviously will experience his relationship with that worker much more positively than the relationship with the other workers. But does this mean that the *laissez faire* worker has a "better" relationship than the others? Better in what sense? Will it yield better learning and growth for the child? Is it a less conflict-ridden relationship but one that may teach the child some wrong things? Will that worker be able to deal with tough issues with the child once the child is used to getting an "easy ride" from the worker? Is the child losing out on other possible relationships because the relationship with the *laissez faire* worker biases the child against the other workers? Conversely, is a relationship featuring a great deal of conflict and hardship necessarily a bad one? Is it better to have no relationship at all than to have one that is conflict ridden?

Given all of these questions (none of which have a *right* answer), how meaningful is the statement, "I have a good relationship with little Eric?" What does it actually tell us about Eric, about how to work with Eric, and about how Eric might be experiencing his time in the program?

Let us look at the second statement: "Eric has trouble forming relationships." Presumably what we are observing is that Eric is not talking much with any of the staff, mostly does his own thing, perhaps is aloof and quiet, and generally seems alienated from the program. This may lead us to conclude that he is having trouble forming relationships. But is this a fair conclusion? We can consider some other possibilities. Could it be that the way in which we are approaching the development of a relationship with Eric simply does not appeal to him? Or maybe he feels that by positioning himself at some distance from the staff he is expressing his experience of the relationship he has with those staff. It may also be possible that Eric really wants to have a relationship with some staff but worries about how that might impact the staff he does not want to have a relationship with. Does Eric have relationships outside of the staff group that he feels might be compromised or adversely impacted if he also forms relationships within the staff group?

It is of course impossible to know exactly the degree to which these possibilities might be relevant or present. What we do know, however, is that our perception of Eric's capacity for relationships may significantly impact the work we do with him. Given that we typically view the presence of a relationship as the foundation for everything else, does that mean that in the absence of a relationship we do nothing? Why would it not mean that? Or does it mean that in the absence of a relationship, we switch our approach from a relationship-based approach to child and youth work to some other approach, like a compliance-based approach?

In the third statement, "I have spent some one on one time with Eric to build a relationship with him," we are describing a method of developing a relationship with a child. One-on-one time is almost always seen as conducive to the development of relationships. That seems obvious enough, but even in this statement, we can expose a number of assumptions that may not be entirely valid. One often comes across situations where a child identifies as his or her most significant relationship the one with a worker who sees the child perhaps once every two weeks or even less (this is often the scenario with Children in Care and their Children's Services Workers). This invariably is bothersome to child and youth workers who spend considerably more time, including one-on-one time, with the child. If one-on-one time is the basis for relationship development, how can the child identify someone who he barely sees as more important?

One of the assumptions that we often make about relationships is that their quality is somehow related to the effort we put into it: the more effort, the higher the quality and the more important the relationship. This omits a very important component of relationships inasmuch as it assumes that relationships have meaning outside of their social and emotional context. The social context of relationships is particularly important. To a child (and to adults too), the social standing of the person offering a relationship is extremely important. For example, a movie star taking the time to correspond with a child in a group home three or four times a year may be a much more important relationship for that child than the primary worker in the group home spending one-on-one time with that child weekly.

This may help us remember that relationships do not just unfold through the actions that go into them, but also through the imagination that carries them. The movie star example may be obvious, but the same kind of dynamic can be extended to anyone. Some children and youth feel much more *connected* to a child and youth worker who spends relatively little time with them simply based on how they observe that worker in the context of program activities. If a child admires leadership, a child and youth worker seen to be a leader may have to spend considerably less time with that child in order to *have a relationship* with that child. We bring to our relationships with children not only our actions and our effort, but also our identities and social position within any particular group. This thinking also applies to issues of ethno-cultural heritage, racial identification, gender and spiritual affinity.

Having spend a quite a bit of time rendering complicated what we have thought to be relatively simple, what does all of this mean in terms of language? For one thing, it means that notwithstanding the centrality of relationships in our thinking and in our work, it is very difficult to translate this into language that would adequately address all of the above considerations. Perhaps one lesson is to be careful not to use language that has the potential to trivialize an extraordinarily complex process or concept. The term "relationship" is commonly understood to denote a relatively static *condition*. Moreover, it is a term that implies an emphasis on inter-personal connections, devoid of social and emotional context. As child and youth workers, we know that nothing ever happens devoid of such context and that relationships are not in fact static at all. Quite to the contrary, relationships are a process that is being experienced by all parties to the relationship, and while experiences can be positive or negative, relationships themselves probably are neither good nor bad. If we continue to think in terms of good relationships and bad ones, children and youth who have relationships versus those who do not, and methods of establishing relationships that are based on effort rather than context, we may begin to believe that we have captured the essence of the relationships we might have with any given child or youth. This is always dangerous, because it is entirely possible that this way of "essentializing" relationships is not productive at all. The experience of a relationship for the worker and for the child is probably much more diffuse and may not in fact contain any essence per se.

Engagement

The term "engagement" has increasingly become one of those terms that is easy to use but very difficult to imbue with meaningful content. Does engagement simply mean we talk to kids? Are we talking to them about anything in particular or life in general? And does our engagement of children and youth imply that they are in fact engaged in something? We can relatively easily imagine some very specific circumstances under which the term "engagement" might aptly describe what we are doing. For example:

I engaged Mohamed in conversation.
I engaged the kids in an activity.
I made sure that Mathew is engaged during class time.

In each of the examples above, engagement simply means that we initiated something that involved one or more children or youth. What we asked them to do is what they did. I was talking to Mohamed and he answered my questions, which means that I engaged him in a conversation. Or I told the kids that we will be playing hide-and-seek now, and they went to hide while I was trying to find them; thus, I engaged the kids in an activity.

But let us look more closely at some of the linguistic connotations of the term "engagement." Unlike the phrase "I had a conversation with Mohamed," when we say "I engaged him in a conversation" we are implying that Mohamed was excited about having that conversation. He was not just answering my questions, but it was a conversation that was being carried by both of us relatively equally. Engagement, much like it is used in the context of preparing for marriage, requires that all parties are not just participating but want to participate and are some what excited about it. Imagine asking your partner if she or he would like to be engaged to you and the answer is, "Oh well, I guess so." How would you interpret that? Would you proudly tell everyone that you are now engaged, or would you perhaps wait for a while to see if the enthusiasm steps up a little?

Having a conversation with a child and engaging that child in conversation are not the same thing. Similarly, making children or youth participate in specific activities is not the same as engaging them in those activities. Typically we might say that "I asked the kids to do their chores and they did"; we would not say that "I engaged the kids in doing chores," because we would know that the kids are doing so either because there is a reward (often they earn some allowance) or the consequence for refusing is too great.

Once again it is important to think about what engagement might mean before trying to articulate this to others. If we are truly thinking of engagement as a two-way process rather than simply as a description of our initiatives vis-à-vis the children or youth, then we may have to ponder in a little greater detail the implications of the term.

If engagement is a process, we might want to start by asking where this process begins. Is it our initiative in doing something or is there a prior step. One might argue that since engagement requires that the child or the children are enthusiastic or at least interested in whatever it is we are about to do, the first step is to think about who the child is, what the broader context of our coming together with this child is, and what the specific context we currently face might be. Engagement is not or at least ought not to be a random process but, instead, it should be one that is strategic and targeted. The decision to engage is in and of itself a significant moment in our coexistence with the child since we spend far more time disengaged. We might want to consider what the child will think when we initiate a conversation or a particular activity:

> *You've been sitting in the office for the past two hours; why are you approaching me now?*
>
> *Why should I engage with this person who I barely know?*
>
> *The last time I allowed myself to get sucked into a significant conversation with this dude, he told everyone my deepest secrets; why in the world would I do that again?*

Children and youth are—and ought to be—cynical of our intentions. Most of the time, our intentions are to get them to do something they really do not want to do: get out of bed, do a chore, do their school work, be nicer to others, go to bed, be respectful. Therefore, to be engaged with a child and youth worker is counterintuitive through the eyes of the child or youth. Sure, they might respond to what we are asking, and sure, they might even do what we are telling them to do, but this is hardly reflective of engagement. So what is the meaning of engagement? What is it that we are engaging about? And how do we think about engagement so as to capture the answers to the above questions?

Perhaps the meaning of engagement is to provide the children or youth with an opportunity to voice their thoughts about whatever it is they wish to voice their thoughts on. And, if that is the case, then the process of engagement can best be seen as one of exploration. Specifically we, as the initiators of this process, are exploring what might be of interest and importance to the children and youth we are trying to engage. This changes the concept a little from the simple idea of starting a conversation with a child. Now we are merely the initiators of the process of engagement, while the sustainability of the process and its evolving meaning is really driven by the child! As Batsleer (2008, p. 77) put it, "Conversation that engages young people's interest and moves into new kinds of opportunities and activities is the purposeful conversation of youth work. It is a dialogue which enables information-giving and offers choices about the direction and participation to the young person." Perhaps this is one of the reasons why very control-oriented child and youth workers have such a difficult time engaging children or youth; it is tough to initiate something without controlling where it might go!

Henry Maier (2007) once talked about this in one of his practice hints. He was describing a shift in a group home for younger children who were bored and seemingly demoralized. Maier describes watching a staff member tossing a pillow at one of the children in a playful manner. This is an example of initiating the process of engagement. The staff member had no way of knowing how the child might respond, much less how the other children might feed into whatever the response might be. But she did so anyway, and as it turned out, the child responded by tossing the pillow at another child, who in turn tossed it back at the staff. Before long, the children picked up all kinds of pillows and a massive pillow fight was underway. The children were engaged in an activity that was initiated by the child and youth worker, but not necessarily envisioned to unfold in this way. She went with where the children took it, and unlike so many other activities that are staff initiated and staff controlled, this one ended up being an activity reflecting the principles of engagement at their best.

I once watched a child and youth worker play a board game with a group of youth in a school setting. Before long, one of the youth yelled profanities at the others, the others responded in kind, and the child and youth worker redirected all of them and insisted they focus on the game. The youth did for a short while and then clearly were losing focus and no longer appeared interested. The worker had to go to the bathroom and another worker stepped in. Again one of the youth started swearing at another one, but rather than redirecting, this child and youth worker said something along the line, "You realize that if you keep swearing at him you give him permission to swear at you." The other youth became very excited at the prospect of being able to swear back with permission and quickly agreed with the staff. Some of the other youth agreed too, while others suggested that they would not take so well at being sworn at. Within about 30 seconds I saw a group of youth disengaged and bored with a board game become re-engaged and quite excited about a discussion pursuant to issues of fair game, dealing with insults, stepping over limits, and resolving conflict.

Once again we have taken a seemingly simple idea that has an obvious meaning in common language and we have made it exceedingly complicated. And once again I would suggest that the reason we have done this is to ensure that our thinking about this core concept of child and youth work is not limited to the obvious language attached to it. The concept is hardly obvious, and we would very likely miss the subtleties of the process of engagement in our thinking and therefore in the way in which we articulate it to others if we do not consider them at some length first. Some of the language challenges that we might run into are exemplified by these kinds of statements about children or youth:

1. *Lars is easily engaged.*
2. *I am a great child and youth worker because I can easily engage kids.*
3. *Kwasi is struggling with the program and I need to find a way of engaging him.*

Here are some plausible paraphrases of these statements; is this what you thought was being said?

1. "Lars easily follows the expectations of the program and he is polite and friendly most of the time." Or, "Lars doesn't really follow any of the rules or any of the activities in the program, but he absolutely loves talking about some things that are of interest to him if you let him; turns out he is quite engaged in issues related to social justice and also some of the conflicts amongst groups of teenagers in the community!"
2. "When I am on shift, kids are busy and they always complete all of the program routines. Even if they don't want to, I find ways of making them, because there is no way that I am going to have kids tell me what the agenda is!" Or, "I have spent a great deal of time listening to what the kids are talking about and watching what they like to do when no one is imposing some other activity on

them. Turns out that they got lots of things that interest them, and I am beginning to think that our program and our expectations are not really useful for this particular group of kids."

3. "I really need to spend more one on one time with Kwasi because if I don't engage him soon around his difficulties with our program he is going to get himself kicked out." Or, "I am not effective in engaging Kwasi through the usual means provided for by the program; we need to explore with him what might be of interest to him."

There are unlimited ways of thinking about engagement and therefore of creating meaning by using the term. What is of importance is that we become more aware of the assumptions we make when we use the term to denote what seems obvious. When it comes to children and youth nothing is ever obvious.

Very much related to language, we should briefly consider the many methods of engagement. For the most part, when we speak of engagement, we picture a verbal exchange between child and youth worker and child. But this too is not at all a reasonable assumption. In fact, given the many reasons children have to be a little tongue shy with us (there usually is a consequence if they say the wrong thing), other methods of communication may yield much better and more substantial processes of engagement. In a residential program in Ontario, one of the child and youth workers came up with the idea of exchanging letters with one of the residents who seemed profoundly disinterested in anything the staff or program had to offer. Although they saw each other face-to-face every day, the child and youth worker and the resident were engaged in dialogue and exploration only by means of exchanging letters two or three times a week. Interestingly, the resident's disposition in the letters was completely different than her disposition in face to face interactions. Where she might have been described as oppositional, lacking in empathy, and generally anti-social in her face-to-face interactions with others, she was enormously insightful, very sensitive and thoughtful in her letters, and quite prepared to take responsibility for her behaviours throughout the week. This type of engagement was effective because the control usually associated with face-to-face interactions was mitigated by removing the immediate threat of repercussions for saying the wrong thing or for saying something in a way that might offend. Instead of repercussions, there were discussions, and out of those discussions came resolutions.

If we were to use the term engagement in speaking to others about what we do, how could we do so without losing some of the subtle meanings discussed above? At a minimum, we should know by now that to simply speak of "engaging kids" is probably not enough. Here are some alternative ways of conveying the ideas discussed above in a reasonably concise manner:

> As a child and youth worker, I use a variety of engagement strategies as a way of ensuring that children and youth are able to find opportunities for speaking their mind, for doing things that interest them, and for exploring things that might turn out to be relevant to them.

> Engagement is one of the core activities of child and youth work and is designed to deepen the connection between worker and child so as to facilitate an ongoing exploration of the child's strengths and competencies.

> It is through the engagement of children and youth that I, as a child and youth worker, can get some immediate feedback about the approaches I am taking in connecting with the kids. Without engagement, I am simply imposing my way of thinking, which may end up contributing to the child's view of him or herself as marginal, irrelevant, or incompetent.

LANGUAGE AND VOICE IN CHILD AND YOUTH CARE PRACTICE

As a "talking profession," we have to remain mindful of what we say and how we say it, but we also want to ensure that our voice is heard when and where it matters. In many practice settings, particularly in schools and in residential programs, child and youth care practitioners often complain about feeling "voiceless"; while they are asked to be present with the child or youth moment-to-moment, when it comes to decision-making or developing plans for that child or youth, the voice of the practitioner becomes secondary to the voices of professionals from other disciplines and often with much more limited roles in the life of the child or youth.

The complaint about voice is legitimate, and practitioners are quite right to argue that marginalizing their voices might not be in the best interest of the child or youth. Complaining, however, rarely results in change, at least not in professional contexts (children might have a different perspective on this). Ultimately in most human service settings, voice is not given; it is taken. And in order to take the child and youth care voice into multidisciplinary and often cross-sectoral case management contexts, the importance of using language carefully and with targeted goals cannot be overstated.

Seeking voice represents a professional issue for child and youth care practitioners in at least two distinctive ways. First, what is at stake is the status of the profession itself. While practitioners may be aware of the skills and knowledge they apply to the work each and every day, careless or uncritical use of language can quickly negate the value of such skills and knowledge by trivializing or at least normalizing what the practitioner does. In relating their work to other professionals, practitioners often fall into the trap of purely descriptive accounts of activities and client behaviors. For example, a practitioner might update a multidisciplinary service team about the client's status over the course of the past month by describing what the client did and how the client reacted at different stages of his program participation. Such information is useful but not at all reflective of the role of the practitioner. It says nothing at all about the context of relationships, the active caring or the experience of engagement between worker and client. In a sense, the practitioner ensures that his role is marginalized in the case management process as one of reporting on client progress rather than as one of active participation in client growth and change. The practitioner's voice is limited to a role of information-provider. With some attention to language, the practitioner can generate much greater opportunity for voice. What child and youth care practitioners do is integrally related to how children and youth experience their service (treatment, the program or the intervention), and therefore it is directly related to case management concerns.

The other way in which seeking voice represents a professional issue for practitioners relates to the accuracy of how the client is perceived by the team of professionals who all have varying degrees of knowledge, contact and relationships with that client. One of the core benefits of using the discipline of child and youth care in facilitating change and growth for children and youth is the life space orientation of the discipline. In practice, it is almost always the child and youth care practitioner who can most effectively speak to the impact of services on clients within their life spaces. Most other professionals involved are able to receive feedback about their work only in the context of preset meetings or the artificial spaces of offices, clinics or institutions. The need for voice is therefore not just about the professional ambition of practitioners, but it is also about ensuring that practitioners can actually do their job. Without voice, child and youth care practice is relegated to supporting the implementation of recommendations from individual or groups of professionals working with incomplete information. Again, therefore, it is necessary for the practitioner to ensure that the language through which information is conveyed to others is carefully chosen, does not convey unexamined truths, and does not contribute to superficial or peripheral conclusions about children and youth in terms of their capacities, their identities or even their prognoses.

REFERENCES

Batsleer, J. R. (2008). *Informal learning in youth work*. London: SAGE.

Casson, S. (2005). Developing a shared language and practice. *Child and Youth Services, 27,* 117–149.

DeGenaro, W. (Ed.). (2007). *Who says: Working class rhetoric, class consciousness and community*. Pittsburgh, PA: University of Pittsburgh Press.

Fewster, G. (2005). I don't like kids! *Relational Child and Youth Care Practice, 18*(3), 3–5.

Fox, L. (1994). The catastrophe of compliance. *Journal of Child and Youth Care, 9*(1), 3–18.

Maier, H. (2007). Genuine child care practice across the North American continent. *CYC OnLine*, Issue 104(September). Retrieved January 31, 2009, from http://www.cyc-net.org/cyc-online/cycol-0709-maier.html

Perry, S. (2006). *Words, values and Canadians: A report on the dialogue at the national symposium on language*. Vancouver, Canada: Centre for Addictions Research of BC.

Samovar, L. A., Porter, R. E., & McDaniel, E. R. (Eds.). (2007). *Communication between cultures*. Belmont, CA: Thompson/Wadsworth.

Sayer, T. (2008). *Critical practice in working with children*. New York: Palgrave Macmillan.

Suderman, J. (2007). *Understanding inter-cultural communication*. Toronto, Canada: Thomson Nelson.

Professional Development and Career Building in Child and Youth Care

SUMMARY. This article explores the current status of professional development within the child and youth care field. Pre-service, in-service and professional development activities and systems are critically examined in residential and nonresidential contexts, and barriers to more effective training within the field are identified. While there has been considerable effort both in terms of research and practice with respect to pre-service curriculum development, it is argued that in-service training for practitioners is sparse, often random and rarely coordinated to meet the knowledge and skill needs of practitioners relative to their specific employment context. Foundational elements for career building in child and youth care are also explored, and it is argued that notwithstanding virtually unlimited opportunities for career building and the expansion of the field, there are some areas of practice that are beyond the scope of the child and youth care profession. Particular emphasis is placed on some of the contradictions between child and youth care theory and practice fields such as child protection, therapy and diagnostic work.

KEYWORDS. Career building, child and youth care training, child and youth workers, child protection, diagnostic work, pre-service curriculum, professional development, residential care, therapy

One might intuitively assume that the foundation of the practitioner's knowledge and skill is built through the pre-service training that practitioner completes. By "pre-service training" I mean the formal educational programs that a practitioner completes before entering the field. And yet we know that this assumption has its flaws: For one thing, many individuals currently serving the functions of child and youth care have never completed any pre-service training. Recent estimates in Ontario, Canada, for example, are that about 50% of current residential child and youth workers do not have a child and youth care diploma or degree; many have alternative certificates in the human services and some have no postsecondary education at all (Stuart & Sanders, 2008). These statistics are based on the child and youth care workforce in a geographic jurisdiction that has a greater concentration of postsecondary child and youth care diploma-granting institutions than anywhere else in the world. Although there are no reliable statistics, one can presume that in other jurisdictions, particularly outside of Canada, the percentage of child and youth workers without any formal child and youth care pre-service training is even greater. While in Canada, at least, education and hospital-based child and youth care practice give somewhat greater consideration to child and youth care specific pre-service training, community-based practice and, in particular, family-focused practice typically has no specific requirements with respect to child and youth care practitioners' pre-service training.

This has a significant impact on considerations for professional development in our field. Under circumstances where there are no specific commonalities in the pre-service preparation of practitioners, it would not be very responsible to rely on the pre-service curriculum for preparing individuals to practice child and youth care; for many, training and professional development starts with being hired by an organization that provides services to children and youth. In and of itself this would not be particularly problematic if we could rely on employers providing all of their employees in child and youth care roles with the conceptual foundation of the discipline. This, however, is not the case, and as we will discuss further below, the provision of in-service training and the availability of professional development opportunities vary considerably amongst employers. Without such foundation, the practitioner's understanding of core concepts such as, for example, "caring," "relationship," "engagement," and "life space intervention" are formed through the interpretation of day-to-day events and occurrences, disconnected from theory and the conceptual context of these concepts. It is not surprising, therefore, that while the majority of practitioners can reference the core concepts of the discipline, a considerably smaller number can do so in a way that corresponds to their intended meanings. In the following discussion, we will consider some of the core themes related to professional development in our field. As a result of the dominance of the residential context in which our field has developed, we will first examine training and professional development in relation to residential child and youth care, and then expand our thinking to other settings and contexts where child and youth care practitioners might work. Before proceeding, however, it is useful to define some of the terms related to training and professional development used throughout the article.

TRAINING TERMINOLOGY IN CHILD AND YOUTH CARE PRACTICE

Mirroring the inconsistencies in training practices throughout the children and youth services sector, the language used to describe specific aspects of human resource development in the field of child and youth care practice varies not only between geographic jurisdictions but even amongst employers within the same geographic jurisdiction. In order to avoid confusion, therefore, I will limit myself to the following terms that describe various stages and aspects of child and youth care practitioner training.

Pre-service training

Pre-service training refers to the formal educational qualifications pursued by practitioners prior to entering the field; typically this involves completion of a post-secondary diploma or degree and, in practice, it may involve the completion of an educational program that is specific to the discipline of child and youth care practice or it may involve the completion of a wide range of "relevant" educational programs ranging from professional certificates, diplomas and degrees in social services to more generalist university degrees in traditional academic disciplines such as sociology or psychology.

Orientation training

Orientation training refers to the initial preparation required of a practitioner when entering a particular work place. Orientation is typically offered as a standardized process designed by the employer to ensure that the practitioner is sufficiently familiar with day-to-day responsibilities. While some employers provide extensive orientation for practitioners, that includes an orientation to the agency and all of its activities, other employers provide relatively brief orientations focused on the specific activities the practitioner will likely be engaged in as he starts his employment in the organization.

In-service training

In-service training refers to the training that practitioners receive once they have been hired into a position with an agency or organization providing services to children, youth and their families. Such training can consist of organizational policies and procedures as well as workshops, seminars or presentations about specific elements of typical client profiles (such as Fetal Alcohol Spectrum Disorder [FASD], psychiatric disorders, behavioral patterns), developmental themes (such as attachment theory), or specific approaches to working with children and youth such as "collaborative problem solving," "play therapy," or "cognitive-behavioral therapy."

Mandatory training

Mandatory training refers to specific certifications or skills that every practitioner in a given service context must have as a result of legislative or regulatory requirements within a particular jurisdiction and can include crisis intervention strategies, medical emergency intervention skills and demonstration of knowledge about policies and procedures. Such training is most commonly mandated within the residential context of child and youth care practice. Mandatory training can also include specific knowledge or skills the employer deems essential and requires of all of its employees. Increasingly common examples of this type of non-legislated but nevertheless mandatory training include "diversity" or "cultural competency" training, training related to major legislative changes relevant to the employer's work, or specific activities that relate to the organizational culture the employer would like to foster or promote.

Professional development

Professional development refers to learning opportunities accessed and activities carried out by practitioners that may not be specifically related to the current employment context but that more generally advance or enhance the skills and knowledge of the practitioner within the children and youth serving sectors. Examples of professional development can range from workshops and seminars about alternative ways of working with children and youth, to registration in formal educational programs that relate but are not specific to the current employment context (such as pursuing a graduate degree in psychology or a professional degree in child and youth care practice, education or social work). Professional development activities are geared toward the career development aspirations of the practitioner more so than the specific circumstances of the practitioner's current work. Professional development most commonly takes place outside of the current employer's in-service training offerings, but could also be combined with such offerings especially in multi-service agencies or organizations.

Career development

Career development refers to the way in which a practitioner envisions his professional future, whether this entails a more clinical involvement with clients or more policy or management-oriented activities in the broader sector of children and youth services. As such, career development is closely linked to professional development, but these two terms are not identical. Whereas the former refers to the specific activities carried out by the practitioner—often not necessarily connected or systematically selected activities—career development refers to the structure or plan in place to support the practitioner moving from one professional activity to another, typically with expectations of greater material rewards and increased correspondence to personal and professional ambitions.

TRAINING AND PROFESSIONAL DEVELOPMENT IN RESIDENTIAL CHILD AND YOUTH CARE

Training and professional development have long been thought of as necessary elements for maintaining a high quality of care in residential settings. For safety reasons, the regulating bodies for such settings impose various mandatory training requirements for staff and enforce the completion of these through some form of licensing process. There are, however, no common standards or requirements for ongoing professional development across politico-geographic jurisdictions, and training practices vary considerably amongst agencies. In Ontario, the only set standards that apply in residential care environments relate to the mandatory certification in crisis intervention. In the United States, there are some variations across states. However, few states have standards that elevate training and professional development requirements beyond crisis intervention and medical first aid. In Scotland, a greater emphasis on ongoing training and professional development was instituted following several client deaths during the late 1990s and early 2000s, even resulting in the establishment of the Scottish Institute for Residential Care.

The child and youth work literature is replete with studies, articles and editorials about professional development: The bulk of these relates to pre-service activities and makes no reference to in-service professional development. Thus, Forkan and McElwee (2002), Krueger (2005), Phelan (2005), and Shahariw Kuehne and Leone (1994) examine the current state of pre-service curriculum at both college and university levels in some detail. Likewise, Beker and Maier (2002), Clarini and Greenwald (2004), and Vaughan (2005) have been commenting on the specific requirements of pre-service training and professional development for child and youth work positions in Canada, the United States, the United Kingdom, and Australia. Kobolt (2005), Vaughan (2004), and Romi (2001) have provided evaluations and international comparisons of pre-service training approaches for Slovenia, Australia, and Israel respectively. Jacobs (1995) details the development of pre-service curriculums in Scotland in the mid-1990s.

In addition to studies about the pre-service training curriculum for child and youth workers, there are a number of research studies about the types of skills and competencies required by the field itself. Thus, Stuart and Carty (2006) recently completed a study of essential competencies for residential child and youth workers in the Children's Mental Health sector of Ontario, as identified by supervisors active in the sector. The seven competencies identified in their study speak to the ever-deepening and increasingly more complex roles of child and youth workers. Recognition is given to participation in integrated case management practices, multi-disciplinary case conferencing, and the development and implementation of treatment plans.

Similarly, Garza, Borden, and Astroth (2004) co-edited an issue of *New Directions for Youth Development* that details youth worker professional development themes and approaches in the United States. Amongst the core themes cited in this volume is the necessity of professional development as the "cost of doing business" (Quinn, 2004) and the benefits of systematizing professional development activities across agencies and even sectors (Johnson, Rothstein, & Gajdosik, 2004). Much like Stuart and Sanders (2008), Astroth, Garza, and Taylor (2004) also identify core competencies required to work effectively in the field, and their list corresponds closely to that of Stuart and Sanders.

In spite of the commonly held view that ongoing training and an emphasis on best practice are essential components of good child and youth work, there has been relatively little attention paid on what type of training child and youth workers receive once they are employed in the field. As mentioned, most residential child and youth workers are required to take a range of certification trainings annually, including training in crisis intervention and physical restraints, First Aid and CPR, as well as training related to agency policies and procedures, health and safety and fire safety. Beyond that, however, there are no regulated standards for professional development in the field. Essentially, the availability of training opportunities is usually at the discretion of the agency and, perhaps, the professional network or association in which they participate.

A number of scholars have pointed to the importance of ongoing professional development, but there are no current studies of what that might look like. Murphy (1994, p. 32), for example, points out that, "At worst, it is irresponsible, and at best naïve of agencies to believe that staffing residential programs with inexperienced, untrained or under-trained staff will somehow benefit clients." Kiraly (2001, p. 123) argues that "In-service training is an investment for an agency. The creation of a learning environment in the workplace is a key component of delivering quality service. . . ." Her analysis suggests furthermore that ongoing professional development is one of the more effective approaches to preventing child abuse by institutional care givers in residential settings.

Cassidy and Kimes Myers (1993) as well as Peterson, Young, and Tillman (1990), while recognizing the importance of ongoing professional development for residential workers, suggest that self-monitoring and mentorship might be the more practicable ways of achieving this. Borden and Perkins (2006) as well as Huebner, Walker, and McFarland (2003) all point to the inadequacies of existing standards with respect to in-service professional development but none provide any data on what actually happens in the field. McAdams and Foster (1999) provide an interesting account of inadequacies of restraint method training approaches and suggest that physical interventions can be prevented through training in broader ecological understanding of the residential context. Again, however, there is no specific data on what training actually does take place in the field. From an entirely different perspective, Finnell (1992) considers in-service training in relation to reducing staff turnover at a particular residential facility in the United States. His work speaks to the importance of providing "orientation" to new child and youth workers (CYWs), and he applauds in particular the implementation of three day retreats during which more seasoned CYWs "train" newly hired ones.

Notwithstanding extensive contributions to the child and youth work literature with respect to training and knowledge generation issues, there continues to be very little research, writing, and even editorializing about the meaning and role of in-service training for child and youth workers. In fact, there is not even an inventory of what in-service professional development for residential child and youth workers might look like. This lack of information is surprising given that most of the codes of ethics currently in place through the various provincial, state and national associations of child and youth workers in Canada and the United States specifically cite the need to maintain currency in best practices and evidence-based approaches as one of the core principles.

These issues have been acknowledged by some writers in the field, albeit without much detail or new information being contributed. Greenwald and Clarini (2001) cited concerns about the nature of connections between pre-service curriculum design and in-service training for child and youth workers in a brief article in one of the major journals of the field. Specifically, they question whether the effort on the part of educational institutions to respond in their curriculum development activities to the needs of agencies is necessarily a good long term move. According to them, the danger is that child and youth workers increasingly are trained to meet the competency and performance requirements of employers but less to join and participate in the fundamental premises of the profession of child and youth work. Thus, while pre-service training related to the service needs of agencies complements in-service training provided by agencies to raise the clinical know-how of child and youth work staff very well, these complementarities do very little to promote the individual worker's allegiance to and identification as a child and youth work professional.

There has been some recognition in the past 5 to 10 years that there is indeed a need to ensure ongoing professional development for child and youth workers beyond the completion of their pre-service training. After several tragic scenarios in Scotland, for example, the Scottish Institute for Residential Child Care was established in 2000. As part of its mandate, this Institute oversees the ongoing professional development activities of certified residential child and youth workers and sets minimum standards of recognized training participation for renewal of certification which is required every two years (Kendrick, 2004, pp. 73–74). Similarly, the North American Certification Project includes provisions for ongoing training requirements of active child and youth workers and sets specific requirements with respect to continuing professional development hours per certification period (Mattingly & Thomas, 2004). Likewise, the Ontario Association of Child and Youth Counsellors has instituted a training requirement annually as a prerequisite for renewal for "certified" and "full professional" members.

Of course, none of these initiatives provide much comfort in terms of ensuring ongoing preoccupation amongst residential child and youth workers with what has been learned as the foundation of the profession in pre-service training. For one thing, many currently active child and youth workers carry the name of the profession only because they fulfill the role commonly perceived as a child and youth worker role; in fact, many do not have any educational qualifications that are specific to the discipline of child and youth work. In addition, the vast majority of child and youth workers currently active in every jurisdiction in North America and countries around the world are not members of any regulating body or association, and therefore would not be monitored by these in terms of their ongoing professional development.

While we still have not delineated what professional development for residential child and youth care practitioners might look like, we can readily identify several barriers that could potentially pre-empt any movement to improving training standards in residential care. Specifically, we can identify barriers that might be categorized as structural/organizational on the one hand, and practitioner-based on the other.

Structural and Organizational Barriers

Residential settings are structured in accordance with required staffing ratios. This simple fact impacts significantly on the opportunities for professional development for individual workers. Unlike in most other employment contexts, when a residential worker attends training, someone else has to take his place, creating what is commonly referred to as a "replacement cost." In nonresidential employment contexts, the training time of professionals is incorporated into their work schedule, and while it may result in a delay of service, there is no real loss associated with such a professional attending training, and therefore there is no replacement cost. This cost increases the cost of training for residential child and youth workers considerably. In agencies where training is provided and paid for by the employer, this extra cost is accrued by the employer. In settings where the employer does not cover the time of the child and youth worker to attend the training, the extra cost is accrued by the child and youth worker in the form of lost income. Regardless of who ultimately pays for the replacement cost of the child and youth worker, single day or even multiday training events are costly endeavors and often simply do not happen.

Aside from the cost involved in sending residential child and youth workers to training, there are also scheduling implications. Many residential settings experience very unstable scheduling arrangements, whereby full-time workers unable to work due to vacation time, sick time or training time are replaced with casual relief workers. Maintaining a stable list of such casual workers is a challenge for many employers, and even where such lists exist, there is no guarantee that a relief worker will be available for the specific shift needed by the worker to be available for the training event.

Both replacement costs and scheduling issues are exacerbated by the time required to complete training that is considered mandatory by licensing standards or some other regulatory authority. Crisis intervention training, first aid/CPR, and other safety-related trainings that must be completed annually already produce significant costs and scheduling challenges for the employer. Adding further professional development opportunities to this list is therefore often greeted with less than enthusiasm by the employer.

Aside from the structural barriers discussed above, there are also barriers to the professional development of the residential child and youth worker that are based on organizational culture and priorities. In multiservice organizations employing professionals from a variety of disciplines, the professional development of the child and youth worker is often considered secondary to that of other professionals. This is particularly the case where other professionals can lay claim to more extensive regulation on the part of professional associations or regulatory colleges. To some degree, this may also reflect an organization's biases in favor of the more established professions of psychology, social work and even educational staff such as teachers and educational assistants.

In larger organizations, training budgets are commonly centralized, and spending priorities for training events are therefore subject to the above-mentioned biases. Given that child and youth workers almost never manage the budgets associated with training, they are often significantly disadvantaged in settings where they are considered a low-status profession. In addition, multiservice organizations often develop training plans and schedules that child and youth workers can access but that are not necessarily geared toward the learning needs of residential child and youth care practice. In the child welfare sector, for example, all agency personnel may be able to get training in the latest protection standards or legislative amendments to child protection law but the relevance of such training tends to be much greater for individuals working in different roles. The reverse is almost never true: To the extent that there are training opportunities that relate specifically to living with children or youth in a residential setting, other professionals rarely attend. This says a lot about the broader professional estimation of the importance of residential child and youth care.

Finally, organizations sometimes create barriers for child and youth worker access to relevant professional development opportunities inadvertently. Although this is always well-intentioned, many organizations add to the mandatory training requirements for child and youth workers several days of training reflecting organizational priorities. Over the course of the past 10 years, for example, agencies across North America have been adding multiday training events related to cultural competency and diversity to the list of mandatory trainings for all agency staff. While such training may well be beneficial and useful for residential child and youth workers, the added replacement costs and scheduling challenges emanating from such additional mandatory training requirements are rarely taken into consideration.

Practitioner-level Barriers

Child and youth care practitioners themselves sometimes add to the barriers for their own professional development. For many, identifying training needs and opportunities ranks a distant last on the list of professional priorities. In residential settings, promoting training in areas of day-to-day work may also imply admitting to weakness or vulnerability in those areas, which is not something child and youth workers like to do. Unless it is pointed out by a supervisor, many child and youth workers are not likely to publicly admit to feeling challenged by the concept of engagement, or to be struggling with developing relationships with children or youth.

Initiative in terms of professional development is not typically fostered in agencies (it is often promoted as a "good idea," but less often followed up with resources) and therefore individual practitioners frequently do not seek out useful opportunities for learning. In addition, in many residential settings, particularly in the private sector, training is not funded by the employer at all, and as a result, few child and youth workers are prepared to sacrifice their income or their own time and financial resources to invest in training events.

In the specific context of professional development for residential child and youth care practitioners, then, we can summarize the dilemmas pursuant to developing a good training program as follows:

- Inconsistencies in the pre-service qualifications of individuals hired into child and youth work positions;
- Potential gaps in what skills and abilities employers within the field are looking for and what the curricula of colleges and relevant university programs offer;
- Lack of access to training opportunities for child and youth workers in the field;
- Excessive focus on mandatory training requirements at the expense of professional development (especially in residential settings).

PROFESSIONAL DEVELOPMENT IN
NONRESIDENTIAL CONTEXTS

While residential care remains the largest employment context for child and youth workers in North America and likely also in Europe, Australia, and elsewhere, nonresidential employment contexts are proliferating rapidly within the field. In some jurisdictions, such as Western Canada and some U.S. states, residential care has been steadily declining and nonresidential approaches to working with children, youth and families have been growing substantially. In the United States in particular, the phenomenal rise of boarding schools for at-risk youth has resulted in a resurgence of residential child and youth care practice, albeit in a nontraditional (and primarily private) context. In addition to the nonresidential programs where child and youth care practitioners have been working for some time, such as day treatment programs, after-school programs and in schools, today we find practitioners active in hospitals, in the community and especially in family homes. Group work with some type of therapeutic focus is also growing rapidly within the profession, and we now have many child and youth care practitioners providing therapeutic groups to children and youth covering topics as varied as self-esteem, addictions, and pro-social values.

The implications for training and professional development are significant in this context. On the one hand, most pre-service educational curricula have made adjustments to ensure that practitioners receive training and education about at least some of these new employment contexts. Courses about child and youth care approaches to working with families, for example, have been developed in several of the postsecondary institutions providing child and youth care diploma or degree programs. In addition, even in these new and evolving employment contexts, much of the theoretical and conceptual bases of the discipline still remain relevant. Practitioners can, for the most part, draw on their knowledge about boundaries, self, ethics, relationship and engagement and transfer that knowledge to virtually any setting in which they might be working. On the other hand, there is increasingly a discrete body of knowledge and research that applies to particular settings; we can, for example, identify a number of major contributions to working with families that have appeared just in the past five years (Garfat, 2003; Phelan,

2003). The question then becomes how child and youth care practitioners access this material and how they might be exposed to new or newly formulated ways of approaching their jobs?

In most contexts, training and professional development opportunities for practitioners working in nonresidential contexts are in fact available and accessible. Unlike in the residential context, in these new employment contexts child and youth workers are not disadvantaged by the structural barriers to accessing training that we identified earlier. There are, however, a number of barriers to training and professional development that reflect the relative novelty of this employment context for the profession. These include the following:

- Many employers are themselves unsure about how the profession of child and youth care fits with the employment context; the use of child and youth care practitioners is often motivated by the lower salaries compared to social workers rather than by clear contemplation about the discipline itself;
- In many instances, the use of child and youth care practitioners reflects the introduction of a new discipline to an agency or organization; as a result, there are no clear professional development processes in place to support that new discipline and child and youth care practitioners are simply integrated into existing approaches to professional development and training already in place for other disciplines;
- Many nonresidential programs employing child and youth workers are modeled after evidence-based approaches developed elsewhere by other disciplines; as a result, the training and professional development that is offered frequently reflects not so much the day to day approaches of child and youth care practice, but instead the predetermined sequence of activities associated with the evidence base.

All of these barriers paint a bleak picture for the prospects of effective training and professional development opportunities for child and youth care practitioners, both in residential and nonresidential contexts. In fact, the current status of training and professional development is not quite as bleak as it might appear. There have been several important developments that have provided greater access for child and youth care practitioners to remain informed and involved in the knowledge generation and acquisition process directly relevant to their day-to-day experiences. One of the characteristics of these new developments that are promising is the reliance on the initiative of the practitioner, in conjunction with the practitioner's advocacy to ensure that employers provide at least some funding for such initiatives. Examples of such opportunities include the proliferation of local, national, and international conferences that are specific to the field of child and youth care practice as well as the increasing availability of electronic and hardcopy research materials, including scholarly research journals and more accessible "conceptual" journals such as *Relational Child and Youth Care Practice, Reclaiming Children and Youth*, and *CYC On-Line*, a monthly publication on CYC Net.

The concept of self-initiated professional development, therefore, requires that practitioners begin to engage with the resources that are already available and generally accessible and that are reflective specifically of the field of child and youth care. But it certainly does not end there. Learning about child and youth care furthermore requires an ongoing engagement with related professional fields and their knowledge and approaches to providing services. The integration of multiple disciplines in service provision surely is one of the characteristics of contemporary system designs and practitioners must find ways of staying informed about the perspectives and approaches from all the major disciplines.

Beyond attendance at child and youth care conferences and engagement with knowledge and approaches that relate directly to the services in which child and youth care practitioners are employed, there are other professional development activities that can be considered, particularly when we expand our thinking about professional development from its relationship to training and skill building to its relationship to career building. Such activities can include the following:

- Acquiring foreign languages, particularly in large urban work environments;
- Building information technology skills;
- Developing expertise in cultural competency and anti-oppression frameworks;
- Becoming knowledgeable about research and program evaluation;
- Acquiring advanced certifications in wilderness activities;
- Specializing in specific themes related to client trauma, such as sexual abuse, substance use or attachment challenges;

- Developing and demonstrating leadership skills, supervision skills (by becoming a student placement supervisor) and organizational management skills.

The opportunities for professional development and career building are in fact plentiful in our field, but they do require a significant degree of initiative. The standard offers of training and professional development for most child and youth care positions will not, by themselves, open too many doors for career building, and in some cases, they may not even serve the obvious purpose of enhancing the practitioner's capacity to deliver service to children, youth and their families. Although this does vary considerably depending on the employer, waiting for professional development to happen is an insufficient strategy.

Career options for child and youth care practitioners include a wide range of activities and employment contexts, many of which have already been cited through this and previous articles. Increasingly, however, it is viable to consider career options that might not be directly related to practice environments but that can be adjusted to represent "child and youth care practice-informed" approaches to specific activities and positions that have impacted the profession for many years. Examples of such positions include the following policy analysis at local and national government level, scholarly and action research relevant to the field, academic careers in child and youth care, and entrepreneurial initiatives in child and youth care practice.

While the career opportunities for child and youth care practitioners are nearly unlimited, especially when practitioners demonstrate the necessary initiative to pursue professional development activities, there are some career choices that may not be the most appropriate in terms of transferring child and youth care principles to other endeavors. Three such career choices come to mind: child protection work, therapy, and diagnostic work. Whenever a profession evolves quickly and in all directions, it is useful to take stock of what the profession is able to do, and what it perhaps should not try to do. Like all professions, there are limitations, and below we will explore some of these limitations in order to ensure that we remain focused on the ideals of our profession and do not feel pressured to adjust these in order to adapt to new types of assignments.

LIMITATIONS OF CHILD AND YOUTH
CARE PRACTICE

It is important to qualify the term "limitation" somewhat. When we consider the limitations of our profession, we are not necessarily talking about capacity issues. Of course, these too are important issues, and we should always be aware of and honest about the things we are actually trained to do. But beyond capacity, we have to concern ourselves with the theoretical orientation of our profession, its values and ethics, and the language that provides a foundation for just about everything we do. Sometimes, we might want to limit ourselves not because we cannot do something, but because we just do not want to.

PROTECTION WORK IN CHILD WELFARE

The child-welfare sector has been one of the fastest growing employers of child and youth workers in many parts of North America. Child and youth workers in child welfare have taken on a wide range of roles and functions including, of course, residential group care. In a number of child welfare agencies, child and youth workers are employed in residential programs that are hybrids between foster care and group care. Beyond residential services, however, child and youth workers are also working in other capacities for child welfare agencies including family support work (Fitzpatrick, 2008; sometimes called intensive in-home service programs or multisystemic treatment services), various therapeutic groups for children and adolescents, outreach work for older adolescents living on the streets or in the shelter system, and support work for foster homes on a case by case basis. It is certainly fair to say that over the course of the past ten years or so, the profession of child and youth work has found a solid foothold in the child welfare sector (Oliver, 2008). None of these jobs, however, are protection-based jobs. "Protection work" in this context refers specifically to those instances where the child has already been found of an immediate need for protection, or where the worker is actively investigating allegations related to the violation of the child's well being, and a final determination about the risk of harm to the child has not yet been made. Child welfare agencies have, at the core of their mandate, the protection of children. This process unfolds under some very strict legislative and regulatory policies and procedures, and these impact on the nature and scope of flexible decision-making, empowerment work, collaboration, and experiential work. The goal of protection is to ensure that kids are safe in their day to day life, and the work of protection is not designed (quite rightly so) to allow for time as one of the main ingredients of change.

This does not mean that protection workers cannot use their skills and education in their day-to-day tasks. Most protection workers go far beyond the application of risk assessment criteria in making decisions about what should happen next. In fact, it is probably fair to say that the vast majority of protection workers do what they can to develop collaboration and joint decision-making approaches with even the most marginal of families. On the other hand, protection work imposes limits on what can and cannot happen and the degree to which and the length of time that the status quo can remain in place. Beyond that, protection workers invoke the power and control of the courts in order to make sure that kids are safe.

Child and youth care practice as a professional discipline does not lend itself to this type of work for a number of reasons:

- As part of our discipline, we value the concept of experience, which means that in most situations, we are concerned with understanding and making meaning of the things that our clients and we ourselves are experiencing. This approach is very much rooted in the developmental perspective that provides the foundation for our work, but it does not lend itself to an action-oriented framework based on a somewhat formulaic approach to assessing risk and family functioning, often after only minimal observation.
- Child and youth workers work through the medium of relationships. The integrity of our work is very much tied to the integrity of the relationships we develop with clients. This is difficult to maintain under conditions where the threat of court imposed sanctions or consequences is real and may have to be invoked repeatedly.
- The language of child and youth work reflects its focus on experiential work, relationships, and the process of engagement, all articulated through a developmental perspective in which "time" is a major ingredient of change and growth. As for the use of language, our profession seeks to explore the seeds of strength, resilience, and competency even in situations where the indicators of behavior are

overwhelmingly negative and problematic, perhaps even unsafe. It is difficult enough to translate our language in such a way as to assist other professionals to make sense of it. It is enormously difficult, and perhaps not entirely possible, to translate our language into one that meets the criteria of the court process and the requirements of the legal professions associated with this process.

- Finally, protection work requires that engagement with families and children or youth be mixed with an ongoing investigative frame of mind. Even in scenarios where children can be considered safe enough for the time being, the job of the protection worker is to ensure that the level of safety never slips below the threshold of acceptable risk. To do this, no matter what kind of working relationship is established between worker and client, the process of investigation can never stop. Child and youth work, on the other hand, is a profession that is much less concerned about any particular "truth," and instead seeks to develop an understanding of how each person creates meaning for the truth they themselves proclaim, regardless of whether or not any of it is based in fact. Investigation, which really is just another term for "truth-finding," is not a core component (nor a core skill) of child and youth work.

As indicated, then, we have to be careful as child and youth workers not to lay claim to activities or functions just because we are able to do them. Protection work falls outside of the professional and disciplinary goals and ideals of child and youth work, and we therefore have to consider the possibility that this kind of work, interesting and valuable as it may well be, is just not what child and youth workers do or ought to be doing, unless they are able to abandon the core principles of the child and youth care profession and learn and accept those of protection work.

THERAPY

The term "therapy" has long been a confusing one in the human services. Many professions have co-opted it to describe various types of interventions and involvements with clients. Certainly this term is most commonly associated with the counseling professions, but since so many disciplines consider counseling to constitute an integral part of they do, this has not helped much to clarify who actually does therapy, who does not, and who perhaps should not.

In the medical profession, "therapy" often refers to either specific approaches to rehabilitation, such as physiotherapy or occupational therapy or it refers to specific kinds of medication treatments such as chemotherapy, methadone therapy, and pain management therapy. Psychiatrists (also working from a medical model) use the term to refer to various psychotropic drug interventions, including experimental dosages of anti-psychotic medications, mood stabilizers and anti-depressants. Perhaps more closely related to child and youth work is the social work version of therapy. Social workers might use this term to denote marriage or relationship therapy, family therapy, or individual therapy. A little more confusing are situations where the term therapy is attached to a very particular way of promoting growth or development in a child, as in play therapy or even theraplay (a clinical approach to building attachment between child and parent).

Child and youth care practitioners sometimes use the terms "therapeutic" and "therapy" interchangeably. But these are not synonymous terms. Child and youth workers engage clients in therapeutic activities, be that through recreation, play, group conversation, or some other medium (VanderVen, 2003a). Therapeutic activity refers to just about any activity that can be constructed as meaningful from a developmental perspective. This means that virtually anything practitioners do with children or youth can be therapeutic; it really depends on how the activity is used and the child's experience of this activity (VanderVen, 2003a, 2003b). From a child and youth work perspective, therapeutic activity really means thinking about our approaches to a child or youth from within a developmental perspective and trying to ensure that everything we do and say corresponds to the uniqueness of the child or youth, is engaging in the child and youth work sense of that term, and provides opportunities for the child or youth to reflect on some new experiences and make meaning of these in their specific context.

What is perhaps most important when it comes to developing therapeutic activities is that these either take place in the life spaces of the child or youth, or at the very least reflect these spaces and their day-to-day dynamics in some way. The very essence of what we do is to remain focused on our interventions being relevant to the time and place the child can relate to rather than to a setting that reflects the employment context of the "counselor." Moreover, the therapeutic content of our actions comes to life only within the specific relationship that exists between the worker and the child or youth. In fact, our ongoing focus on that relationship is itself a therapeutic activity as a result of which the child or youth can experience him or herself differently.

A simple way of distinguishing the term "therapy" from therapeutic activity is to think of "therapy" as a process that is continuous within the relatively narrow boundaries of the therapy context, whereas therapeutic activity is a process that is continuous within the broader life context of the child or youth. Regardless of how skilled a therapist might be in applying therapy sessions to concrete situations in the person's life, ultimately it falls on the person to experiment with whatever has been learned or thought about in therapy within their own life spaces. The therapeutic activities of child and youth worker and child take place in those spaces to begin with, and therefore whatever is being absorbed by the child or youth is being absorbed in the environment where it is useful.

But therapy is more than this. Therapy also ventures into the very soul of the person engaged in therapy and seeks to explore the meaning of feelings and thoughts through processes of self reflection and guided conversation. In many cases, therapy is issue specific, such as in marriage therapy or family therapy. In all cases, however, really "good" therapy involves a distancing between therapist and client in which the therapist is constantly concerned about un-involving him or herself from the thought process of the client. In other words, therapy is not about joining at all; to the contrary, the therapist offers him or herself as a tool for the client to reflect.

As a result of these dynamics embedded in therapy, child and youth care practice is not a well suited profession to engage in therapy. The concept of distancing is not one that is easily rendered compatible with the child and youth care practice perspective on relationships and their role in worker-client interactions. Moreover, the idea of self-reflection, while critical for the child and youth worker him or herself, is not necessarily a major goal for the client. In fact, the reflective process for the client is explicitly linked to the social, emotional, and systemic contexts of where that client lives his or her life. The comparatively passive tasks of therapy are not ones that meet the core theoretical bases of the child and youth care profession. Our focus on therapeutic interaction and relationships, interestingly enough, almost pre-empts the provision of therapy.

DIAGNOSTIC WORK

This is another common area in which child and youth workers involve themselves without much thought. It happens rather frequently that one hears a child and youth worker speculate on the specific disorder that might be afflicting a particular child. In some cases, the ability to match specific symptoms with a diagnosis is seen as an indication of strong skills and intellectual worth for a child and youth worker. Nothing, however, could be further from the truth. Diagnosing children or youth is well outside of the competency areas of child and youth workers for a number of reasons:

- Pre-service training does not provide a solid foundation for doing so.
- Diagnoses are based on observation and formal testing, and child and youth workers typically are not qualified to administer diagnostic tests. Observation alone sometimes can significantly distort the perception of a client and diagnoses based solely on observation can become a detriment to the client.
- Once a diagnosis has been provided, approaches to a particular client can quickly corrupt the values and methods of the child and youth work profession.

Let us focus for a moment on the last point, because this is a common scenario in many child and youth work setting, especially classrooms and residential programs. It is very important to remember that treatment approaches pertaining to specific diagnoses are not typically developed with the child and youth work profession in mind. In fact, in most cases, such approaches reflect the meta-theoretical content of intervention strategies and are developed paradigmatically in such a way that the specific approaches of various disciplines are neutralized. Cognitive-behavioral therapy or family systems therapy, for example, are two such paradigms that provide fairly explicit instructions on how to work with particular clients.

As child and youth workers, we should, of course, be curious about and interested in such paradigms and their various prescriptions. But this does not mean that we abandon our own theoretical foundation and practice strategies. Whether a child has been diagnosed with ADHD, a conduct disorder, obsessive compulsive disorder, oppositional defiant disorder, an attachment disorder, Asperser's, a mood disorder or anything else, our core principles remain the same: We will care for and about the child by engaging him or her in a therapeutic relationship that takes account first and foremost of the child's humanity, including his or her strength and challenges, within the context of his or her life spaces and identity. None of this means that we must reject the value of diagnostic work altogether. In practice, children, youth, and families living with a diagnosis or even multiple diagnoses incorporate these into their everyday experiences, and therefore, child and youth care practitioners ought to be aware of such diagnoses and approach their clients accordingly. Moreover, child and youth care practice certainly is not one which rejects research and science; there is much to be learned from the research that has been done related to various psychiatric disorders and mental health concerns and, in many cases, there is a substantial evidence base for what types of interventions might work and what types of interventions are best avoided. All of this is critical information for the child and youth care practitioner engaged with children, youth or families who are living with diagnosed challenges; but the practitioner himself should not add to these challenges. Our role in the everyday lives of our clients does not change based on a diagnosis; our specific interventions take account of what we know about the diagnosis and related research, but we continue to work with all the core principles of our discipline.

Disciplinary Limitations and Staying True to the Profession

Many child and youth workers may not like the idea that there are certain things that they just should not do. The "we can do anything" attitude is alive and well within our profession. The desire to do more and hold increasingly more "prestigious" positions is understandable but not particularly useful if it is motivated by a belief that one has learned everything there is to learn about child and youth care. When child and youth care practitioners begin to behave as if they were therapists, social workers or members of some other professional field, children and youth are very likely to lose out. In fact, this is a dangerous attitude to become stuck in. Children and youth deserve to be given opportunities and services that are clear about values, ethics, and disciplinary foundations and orientations. Pretending to be something other than a child and youth worker does not help the profession at all; to the contrary, it takes away from what is really valuable about what we do. Child and youth work has its limitations in terms of how we approach children, youth and families. Once we try to expand beyond those limitations, we run the risk of engaging in activities that are fundamentally about our own ambitions and professional goals rather than the provision of services from a well thought out and increasingly trusted disciplinary framework.

Child and youth care practice can, however, inform other approaches as much as it is informed by these other approaches. It is entirely possible to take on the role of teacher or social worker or even psychiatrist and integrate some of the principles of child and youth care practice into these roles, much like practitioners have been integrating knowledge and skills from other disciplines into their practice. What is important is that the practitioner is clear about the role and mandate of his position. It is inherently a good thing that children and youth experience different adults in different professional roles and different contexts as they make their way through childhood and adolescence. The goal of the practitioner should therefore not be to erase these differences by transferring the child and youth care role into other professional activities. As we seek respect for our discipline, the onus is also on us to be respectful of alternative ways of being with, working with and intervening with children and youth through the core concepts of other discipline and professions. At any rate, the core concepts of child and youth work such as caring, relationships and engagement, are sufficiently complex to keep us interested and excited for some time to come.

REFERENCES

Astroth, K. A., Garza, P., & Taylor, B. (2004). Getting down to business: Defining competencies for entry level youth workers. In P. Garza, L. M. Borden, & K. A. Astroth (Eds.), *Professional development for youth workers* (pp. 25–38). New Directions for Youth Development, *104*.

Beker, J., & Maier, H. (2002). Emerging issues in child and youth care education: A platform for planning. *Child and Youth Care Forum*, *30*(6), 377–386.

Borden, L. M., & Perkins, D. (2006). Community youth development professionals: Providing the necessary supports in the United States. *Child & Youth Care Forum*, *35*(2), 101–158.

Cassidy, D., & Kimes Myers, B. (1993). Mentoring in in-service training for child care workers. *Child and Youth Care Forum*, *22*(5), 387–398.

Clarini, J., & Greenwald, M. (2004). Process and product in designing a new curriculum: The training of special care counselors at Vanier College. *Child and Youth Care Forum, 33*(4), 247–256.

Finnell, S. B. (1992). Reducing child care worker turnover: A case illustration. *Journal of Child and Youth Care Work, 13*, 14–23.

Fitzpatrick, K. (2008). My role as a child and youth worker in child welfare—and why I love it. *Relational Child and Youth Care Practice, 21*(4), 84–85.

Forkan, C., & McElwee, N. C. (2002). Practice placements: A cornerstone for child and youth care training. *Child and Youth Care Forum, 31*(6), 381–396.

Garfat, T. (2003). Working with families: Developing a child and youth care approach. In T. Garfat (Ed.), *A child and youth care approach to working with families* (pp. 7–38). New York: Haworth Press.

Garza, P., Borden, L. M., & Astroth, K. A. (Eds.). (2004). Professional development for youth workers. *New Directions for Youth Development*, 104.

Greenwald, M., & Clarini, J. (2001). Present day concerns about the future training of CYCs. *Journal of Child and Youth Care Work, 16*(2), 298–301.

Huebner, A., Walker, J., & McFarland, M. (2003). Staff development for the youth development professional: A critical framework for understanding the work. *Youth & Society, 35*(2), 204–225.

Jacobs, H. (1995). A new development in the education of direct care practitioners. *Journal of Child and Youth Care Work, 10*, 37–53.

Johnson, E., Rothstein, F., & Gajdosik, J. (2004). The intermediary role in youth worker professional development: Successes and challenges. *New Directions for Youth Development, 104*, 51–64.

Kendrick, A. (2004). Beyond the new horizon: Trends and issues in residential child care. *Journal of Child and Youth Care Work, 19*, 71–80.

Kiraly, M. (2001). Choose with care: A recruitment guide for organizations working with children. *Child and Youth Services, 23*(1/2), 83–124.

Kobolt, A. (2005). An evaluation of training in social pedagogy in Slovenia. *Journal of Child and Youth Care Work, 20*, 83–92.

Krueger, M. (2005). The youth work learning center: Successes and lessons learned. *Child and Youth Care Forum, 34*(5), 357–370.

Mattingly, M. A., & Thomas, D. (2004). The promise of professionalism arrives in practice: Progress on the North American Certification project. *Journal of Child and Youth Care Work, 19*, 209–215.

McAdams, C., & Foster, V. (1999). A conceptual framework for understanding violence in residential treatment. *Child and Youth Care Forum, 28*(5), 307–328.

Murphy, J. (1994). Not just a job: A study of the needs of residential child care workers in Melbourne, Australia. *Children Australia, 19*(1), 27–32.

Oliver, C. (2008). Child welfare work: A life choice, not a life sentence. *Relational Child and Youth Care Practice, 21*(4), 70–78.

Peterson, R., Young, S., & Tillman, J. (1990). Applied ethics: Educating professional child and youth workers in competent caring through self apprenticeship training. *Child & Youth Services, 13*(2), 219–234.

Phelan, J. (2003). Child and youth care family support work. In T. Garfat (Ed.), *A child and youth care approach to working with families* (pp. 67–78). New York: Haworth Press.

Phelan, J. (2005). Child and youth care education: The creation of articulate practitioners. *Child & Youth Care Forum, 34*(5), 347–355.

Quinn, J. (2004). Professional development in the youth development field: Issues, trends, opportunities and challenges. In P. Garza, L. M. Borden, & K. A. Astroth (Eds.), *Professional development for youth workers.* New Directions for Youth Development, 104, 13–24.

Romi, S. (2001). Child and youth care in Israel: Trends and dilemmas in training and in therapeutic intervention programs. *Journal of Child and Youth Care Work, 15/16*, 171–184.

Shahariw Kuehne, V., & Leone, L. (1994). A framework and process for educating students to apply developmental theory in child and youth care practice. *Child and Youth Care Forum, 23*(5), 339–355.

Stuart, C., & Carty, W. (2006). *The role of competence in outcomes for children and youth: An approach to mental health.* Ottawa, Canada: Provincial Center of Excellence for Child and Youth Mental Health.

Stuart, C., & Sanders, L. (2008). *Child and youth care practitioners' contributions to evidence-based practice in group care.* Toronto, Canada: Ryerson University.

VanderVen, K. (2003a). Transforming the milieu and lives through the power of activity: Theory and practice. *Journal of Child and Youth Care Work, 19*, 103–108.

VanderVen, K. (2003b). Overprogramming for the few, underprogramming for the many. CYC OnLine, Issue 57(October). Retrieved January 31, 2009, from http://www.cyc-net.org/cyc-online/cycol-1003-karen.html

Vaughan, B. (2004). Youth worker training: Teaching and learning from an international perspective. *Journal of Child and Youth Care Work, 19*, 192–201.

Vaughan, B. (2005). Youthwork education: A view from down under. *Child and Youth Care Forum, 34*(4), 279–302.

Child and Youth Care Approaches to Management

SUMMARY. This article explores the themes and issues related to child and youth care approaches to management. The profession is significantly underrepresented at the management level. To some extent, this reflects the challenges of being recognized in the broader human services sector as a profession, but perhaps more so, it reflects an underdevelopment of skills, knowledge and managerial pragmatism on the part of the practitioner. It is argued that management customs and requirements place child and youth care values and principles at risk. However, there are steps that can be taken to mitigate such risks. Common themes and processes of management roles are discussed including performance management, orientation, recruitment and supervision. Child and youth care practitioners are ultimately well placed to assume management positions in residential and non-residential contexts but, in so doing, they must ensure that their managerial identity maintains the fundamental values and principles of the discipline.

KEYWORDS. Barriers to management, community-based child and youth care, ethics, human resources, management, middle management, orientation, performance management, recruitment, residential care, supervision, values

With the ever-increasing range of employment opportunities for child and youth care practitioners one can anticipate that there will also be an expanding range of management opportunities. It is perhaps premature to claim that there has already been an increase in the number of child and youth care practitioners in management positions in social service agencies from all sectors. In reality, the dominant sector for child and youth care management positions remains the residential care sector, and even there, management positions are often limited to residential supervisory positions (Ingram & Harris, 2001). In some geographic jurisdictions, notably in Western Canada and some states in the U.S., an increase in community-based approaches to working with youth and families often at the expense of residential care might have resulted in an increase of child and youth care practitioners in managerial positions that are not residential supervisory positions. Another type of program that is commonly supervised by child and youth care practitioners is the day treatment program. This is not at all surprising, since day treatment in many agencies is very closely linked to residential programs, and frequently, the residential supervisor also supervises day treatment programs operated by the same agency. We can, of course, identify many other specific programs that might be supervised by a child and youth care practitioner, but this is not reflective of a trend in the field; more typically, it is reflective of serendipitous circumstances specific to a particular program or agency. As Bracey (2007, p. 25) notes, "Youth services are full of accidental leaders. Very few people I've come across entered the profession because of a driving ambition to lead it. For many, it 'just sort of happens.'"

It is difficult to know precisely why child and youth care, as a profession, has not been successful at breaking into the ranks of management in the human services. Perhaps it relates to somewhat of an aversion to the very concept of management: "The ideas of leadership and management are controversial across the helping professions. In many areas of the public and voluntary sectors discourses of leadership have become associated with 'managerialist' concerns with control, target setting and the measurement of performance.... Those who work with young people often see themselves as advocates for and activists on behalf of the young people they work with, taking their side against the forces of authority..." (Harrison et al., 2007, p. 2). One might speculate that the comparatively lower educational standards for the profession might contribute to this trend. While social workers typically have at least an undergraduate university degree, child and youth care practitioners have a wide range of pre-service educational qualifications that often do not include a university degree. This has, in the past, lead to a call for higher levels of education for practitioners in the field (Ferguson, 1982; Linton & Fox, 1986; VanderVen, 1998). The low status of the profession may also contribute to this trend. For many social service managers, the day-to-day activities of child and youth care practitioners still appear as quite basic, based on intuition and common sense rather than any particular field of knowledge or skill set. While it is easy to blame the ignorance of others for the profession's moderate fortunes in management, it is perhaps also necessary to examine common limitations of practitioners and how these might create barriers in terms of successfully competing for management positions with professionals from other fields.

Without a doubt one such limitation relates to professional communication skills, both written and verbal. While there are many practitioners who have advanced skills in this area, there are far more who do not. The inability to articulate the work of child and youth care practice in clear, concise and professionally relevant language constitutes a major barrier to the career advancement of many practitioners. As long as terms such as boundaries, relationships and engagement are used in ways that fail to convey the complexity of the child and youth care approach, it is unlikely that social service agencies will recognize the management potential of child and youth care practitioners.

Also unhelpful is that many child and youth care practitioners have little interest in the broader themes and issues of their service sector. Funding issues, the complexities of policies and regulations impacting service considerations, and the nuances of program development and evaluation often escape the practitioner entirely, which constitutes a major deficit in terms of management potential. Ascendancy into the ranks of management requires a much broader knowledge base of not only day-to-day service considerations but also of the professional, political and regulatory context of the service itself (Ingram & Harris, 2001). It also requires a thorough understanding of how the multidisciplinary pieces of service delivery fit together, what the issues are in terms of multidisciplinary collaboration, and what the opportunities are in terms of program development, service expansion, partnership development and so on. Management is not ultimately about service delivery; instead, managers provide the foundation of organizational culture, process and procedures related to all of the core areas of agency life including human resources, finances, external relations, policy development and liaison with funders and government or, in the private sector, with customers. Some of the core skills that are required to function effectively as a manager are decision-making, problem-solving, consensus building, analytical skills, risk management skills and, perhaps more so than anything else, the power (or art) of persuasion.

It is precisely because of this list of required skills that I would argue that child and youth care practitioners are ideally suited for management positions in the social services. After all, in their day-to-day work with children, youth and families, child and youth care practitioners are analyzing situations and scenarios at all times. They make decisions while managing risks and they solve problems and build consensus around potential solutions all the time. The challenge for practitioners seeking management positions is to convince other managers that these activities are analogous to what managers do and the skills entailed in completing these activities are transferable to the management sector. This requires an understanding of what management is all about and the ability to articulate this clearly and in a compelling manner.

In this article, we will explore some of the core components, issues and themes that might confront managers in child and youth care environments. A manager in a child and youth work employment environment faces a wide range of challenges for which there often are no easy answers, or even right or wrong answers. Managing anything is frequently about balancing opportunity with known shortcomings. As we explore the professional issues of management, we will try and contemplate what the profession of child and youth care might bring to the job and how the principles of the profession might impact the way in which some of the routine tasks of managers are undertaken. Since the vast majority of management opportunities for child and youth care practitioners are at the program supervisory level rather than the executive management level of social service agencies, we will begin this exploration there. Specifically, we will consider three components of program management that are standard challenges for child and youth care supervisors. These management components are recruitment, orientation, and performance management. Given that all child and youth work based programs are primarily relying on the skills and abilities of their child and youth workers, these three components often turn out to take up the vast majority of the manager's time and energy (whereby the other activity that takes up an extraordinary amount of time especially in residential settings is of course scheduling).

RECRUITMENT

Just because child and youth work is a great profession does not mean that everyone working in our profession is good at what they do. In fact, many are not particularly good at being child and youth workers at all. Although these individuals typically know that they are not so good at the job, they stick around perhaps because no one else in the field would hire them or, alternatively, they have no transferable skills for seeking meaningful employment outside of the field (Gharabaghi, 2005). A manager in any field is only as good as the people doing the work day in and day out. In the field of child and youth care practice, this can pose particularly great challenges, since staffing issues not only impact the goals and objectives set by the manager or the organization, but these issues also affect the well being of children and youth, sometimes with serious long term consequences.

As far back as 1957, Betty Flint observed some of the challenges associated with staffing issues in a residential context, and she described her observations as follows:

> When Miss Kilgour had been appointed supervisor, she had inherited a staff which ... was too busy operating the institution to be aware of the importance of the emotional needs of the children. The staff had been concerned with the comfort of adults, geared to a routine enforcing physical cleanliness, and pleased by any quietness on the part of the children, since quietness was often construed as "goodness." Any child who demonstrated healthy qualities of rebellion or who showed sufficient initiative to make insistent demands on the staff was discouraged by being punished.... Thus, needs of the staff had frequently taken precedence over the needs of the children, and the whole organization depended on arrangements made for the staff's convenience. (1966, p. 33)

Mark Krueger similarly raised concerns about the quality of staffing in residential care in particular. His position reflected a critical view of the system designed to offer services to troubled youth, in which the care givers invariably were secondary to the more established professions (such as psychiatry and social work), and therefore did not benefit from investment in compensation or training and professional development (Krueger, 1986). It was in response to this observation that Krueger began to promote the "team approach" to care giving, in which the disciplinary hierarchies of professional designations are eliminated.

In spite of repeated warnings that the quality of care givers in youth-serving systems was inadequate, not too much has changed over the past twenty or thirty years. In reality, while there are many organizations that have placed much greater emphasis on human resources and human resource development, there are at least as many that have not done so. The result is a rather turbulent mix of staffing types, pre-service qualifications, and in service training provisions. Recent research in Ontario, Canada has shown that only about 40% of care givers in residential programs for children and youth have specific pre-service qualification that match the job at hand (Stuart & Sanders, 2008).

Knowing that not everyone who has the pre-service qualifications for the job is actually going to turn out to be great, the pressure is on the recruitment process to attract enough qualified candidates to be able to choose only the ones that clearly are skilled, motivated, and who share a particular philosophical and value-based disposition. This is easier said than done. The first challenge relates to the type of job being offered, particularly the schedule and the material compensation that comes with it. Also of significant relevance is whether or not the position is a permanent one with benefits or a contract position that may have some extra pay in lieu of benefits but that typically offers no job security whatsoever.

Whereas twenty years ago the material compensation packages for child and youth work positions were relatively balanced throughout the field (nobody was paid well), today, there are significant differences in pay and the scope of benefits that reflect different sectors and even different service providers within the same sector. In Canada, for example, hourly rates for child and youth workers can vary from between $10 to $12 in privately owned and operated group homes, some shelters, and some grassroots outreach programs on the lower end to up to $30 in some hospitals, some school boards, and even some child welfare-operated group homes. Benefit packages also vary considerably, with some employers offering only the mandatory two week vacation, a handful of sick days, and minimal health benefits while others are offering up to five weeks vacation, unlimited accumulation of sick days, short term and long term disability, as well as 100% coverage for most extended health benefits, including the all important dental and drug plans. Some agencies even offer top up pay for parental leaves! Needless to say, for a manager in an urban environment where there are multiple service providers representing multiple sectors, part of the recruitment strategy will have to take account of the competition for experienced child and youth workers. A manager for an employer that is unable to offer a particularly competitive compensation package may have to develop a recruitment strategy that is prepared for high turnover rates.

As important as compensation packages are in the recruitment process, often even more important is the schedule. In general, it is much easier to recruit for day programs that operate Monday to Friday than it is to recruit for a 24-hour environment that operates seven days a week, with a shift schedule that has people working at least day and evening shifts, and sometimes also overnights. The reality is that many experienced child and youth workers are at the stage in life where starting a family is high on the agenda, and shift work just is not conducive to family life. Conversely, many younger child and youth workers or those who have been around for a while but do not have a family typically grow tired of a shift schedule primarily because they find themselves working when their friends are not, and they find themselves not working when many of their friends are.

All of this can serve to reduce the pool of qualified applicants for openings that become available. If the job offered is not all that attractive, there will likely be higher turnover of staff and fewer qualified applicants to meet the manager's needs. It often becomes apparent early in a child and youth care practitioner's management career that the idea of only hiring child and youth workers with the appropriate diploma or degree is not that easy to implement. Especially in an urban environment where there is no local college with a child and youth worker diploma program, but there are several service providers competing for child and youth workers, the dilemma of wanting the right people but needing to fill vacancies as soon as possible arises quickly. Not filling the vacancies may end up burning out the few qualified people left.

Recruitment is an extraordinarily time consuming activity. Aside from posting jobs and ensuring that the posting is available wherever it might be useful, reviewing resumes as these come in, short listing some candidates, scheduling them for interviews, conducting the interviews, and then checking two or three references for every person of interest can take hours and hours and is a process that can extend over a period of days and sometimes weeks. Depending on the specific scenario and the geographic location, there can be a significant delay between a position becoming vacant and a new hire being ready to take on the role. The leaving employee typically is required to give two weeks notice. By the time the posting is up and has been posted for a reasonable amount of time (in a unionized environment this is usually a prescribed amount of time—seven working days would be standard), and interviews are scheduled, the position is usually vacant. Checking references can take several days, following which an offer can be made. Assuming the person accepts the offer, the appropriate documentation must be sought. The most difficult document to get in a timely fashion is the police records check, which in many urban communities can take anywhere from two weeks to eight weeks to receive. Allowing a child and youth worker to work with children and youth before this police records check has been received (in some jurisdictions, it is generally recommended that a "vulnerable persons check" be completed as well, which can take even longer) would be somewhat irresponsible and poor practice, not to mention that it would violate licensing standards in a residential program in most jurisdictions across North America (Kay, Kendrick, Davidson, & Stevens, 2007; Warner, 1992).

Other recruitment related issues a manager encounters fairly regularly include:

Gender balance. Especially in residential programs but also in classroom situations and some specialized community programs, the need for some gender balance within the staff team is often perceived as great. Yet the legal restrictions in place to hire for a specific gender are quite formidable. Given that the vast majority of applicants for child and youth worker jobs are female, achieving gender balance through the recruitment process is quite challenging.

Dealing with foreign qualifications. In larger urban areas, especially those that attract newcomers to Canada or the U.S., one encounters many applicants whose qualifications either are unfamiliar or are of such high caliber that it might seem difficult imagining them doing the work offered.

Ageism. this is one of the more interesting challenges for child and youth workers in management positions. Many applicants (often from other countries) are significantly older than the average child and youth worker in North America. The new child and youth care manager will undoubtedly be tested in terms of his conscious or not-so-conscious biases as to what a child and youth worker should look like.

Excessive workload. Increasingly we are encountering a new phenomenon amongst child and youth workers. Many have not only a full-time job somewhere, but also several part-time or casual jobs. As a manager, one might have two major concerns about this. If a child and youth worker is working 60 to 80 hours a week, how effective can they possibly be in the very complicated and energy-sapping work that is required? And secondly, if a child and youth worker is working for several service providers within the same geographic jurisdiction, issues around confidentiality and ethics become increasingly pertinent. Given the ever-accelerating placement changes for children and youth in recent years, a child and youth worker working in several programs and possibly sectors will likely come into contact with clients as an employee of different agencies. This always begs the question as to what information that child and youth worker can appropriately pass on, and what information would constitute a breach of a child's or youth's confidentiality if passed on to others at another place of employment.

There are countless other issues pertinent to the recruitment process for child and youth workers, however, the ones listed in the preceding paragraphs rank amongst the more interesting ones. Some of these scenarios may be different and many additional scenarios may arise when managing a program in the Far North, or when managing a program with a specific cultural or spiritual affinity. Nevertheless, at this point we will assume that someone has been successfully hired to fill a vacancy, and we will briefly discuss the orientation process for newly hired child and youth workers.

THE ORIENTATION PROCESS

In many employment settings, the first day at work involves some form of orientation to the new workplace, including to safety related issues, physical plant issues and the core policies and procedures of the agency or business. In the human services, this process is surprisingly similar most of the time. In other words, it is a process that takes place because it is necessary to get started, but not because it holds value beyond the logistical considerations it entails. In their 400-page book about developing programs for at-risk youth, for example, Klopovic, Vasu, and Yearwood (2003) devote exactly four sentences to the orientation process! In contrast, I would suggest that the orientation process is a critical component of the child and youth care approach to management, and one that ought to be based on some planning and foresight. For many managers, the orientation process of new staff is something that is easily delegated to some of the more senior front line staff. In fact, given that the orientation process is supposed to orient the new child and youth worker to the children and youth as well as to the program and how it functions, it makes sense to pair that person up with someone who is doing that work day in and day out.

One of the challenges that is often associated with this is that while front-line workers are generally quite capable of showing a new recruit the ropes, explaining who is who and what is what, and demonstrating how paper work is to be completed, they are not as well placed to speak to issues of program philosophy and the fundamental values of the approach that is being aimed for within the particular program. The reason for this is simply that the operational demands of working within a program almost invariably diminish the purity of its philosophical ideals. In other words, if one were to ask all of the front-line staff who have been working in a particular program for some time to describe the philosophy of that program and perhaps the fundamental values associated with it, there is a very good chance that one would receive as many answers as there are respondents.

This has significant implications for the ongoing process of program development. Once we stop talking about philosophy and values, we are very likely to reduce what we are doing to being based either on the idea that "this is how we have always been doing it," or we simply become reactive to the types of situations that we encounter on a day-to-day basis. Thinking about what we do requires hard work and the motivation to remain self critical. When it comes to the orientation process of new recruits, as managers we have to recognize that this is not only a necessity for practical purposes but also an opportunity to refresh the relevance and understanding of program philosophy and values. Every new child and youth worker who joins our program on the one hand has a lot to learn about the specifics of our program but, on the other hand, also has a lot to offer largely because the new team member has not yet been corrupted into the routine of day-to-day problem solving, shift coordination, and trying to just get through.

For this reason, taking some time as the manager to orient new child and youth workers to the program, its philosophy and values, and the expectations related to the core concepts of child and youth work, is time well spent. Of course, all of this raises some questions about what to do when either a new recruit or some of the longer term child and youth workers in the team no longer respond to management direction or no longer work within the fundamental values of the program. The answer to this question will have to come from within the ever unpopular process of performance management.

PERFORMANCE MANAGEMENT

Performance management involves components of many disciplines, including human resources and law, but also social work and counseling, as well as myriad administrative and clerical tasks. We are not going to look at any of these components in great detail as there is far too much to consider to really do any of these themes justice. I do want to provide at least a basic overview of what is involved, because performance management is one of the areas where some of the core principles of child and youth care practice are particularly useful in informing the process.

One of the immediate issues that needs some reflecting on is whether or not there are any specific features of child and youth work in particular that require some adjustment to the more generic, HR-based approach to performance management. I would suggest that indeed, there are such features, and they include the following:

• Child and youth workers work in a very unpredictable environment and the probability of error is great and likely unintended.

- Given the relational nature of the work, so much of a child and youth worker's performance depends on the ability to understand and reflect on "self." This is difficult to measure and can easily lead to violations of human rights and some other loaded scenarios.
- Much like child and youth workers need to reflect on themselves and how this impacts their relationships with children and youth, child youth worker supervisors need to do the same *vis-à-vis* front line workers. Interpersonal conflict or dislike are likely going to distort the supervisor's assessment of the worker's performance.
- A great deal of information about particularly problematic incidents involving child and youth workers often comes from clients, and interpreting such information is not all that easy, given that clients too may have an agenda that is less than pure.
- A great deal of child and youth work is about language and how we "frame" things. Some child and youth workers are very talented in using language and the concept of "framing" as a way of rationalizing very inappropriate actions or inactions.

Certainly this list could be expanded, but many of the scenarios above are ones that I have come across repeatedly as a supervisor and manager. In thinking about performance management within a child and youth work environment, therefore, it is quite critical to remember that this is indeed a *process*, and as such, it can take some time to have a substantial impact on the performance of a particular worker. As a result of this, it is equally important to not miss any opportunities for engaging in performance management. While performance management is indeed a process, it is one that requires the manager's full attention at all times, and one that has to be executed continuously and consistently if it is to have any integrity at all. Here are some basic guidelines to performance management in a child and youth work environment that might be considered by the manager:

- Performance can only be managed if the requirements and expectations about performance are clearly stated and constantly reviewed. Doing so is the responsibility of the manager (or supervisor).
- Philosophically, child and youth work as a profession is committed to strength-based, competency-based approaches that promote resilience and personal growth, all in the context of a developmental perspective. Therefore, the process of performance management

should always have at its core a dialogue about strengths and competence rather than deficits and problems.

- By far the most important tool to ensure that the process of performance management maintains its philosophical integrity is the process of supervision. At an absolute minimum, supervision sessions scheduled with a child and youth worker should be considered high priority by the supervisor and should generally not be re-scheduled to accommodate the supervisor when other meetings come up.
- Performance measures for child and youth workers should reflect the core concepts of the profession in addition to basic employment standards such as attendance and punctuality. If a supervisor is over-focused on basic employment standards at the expense of child and youth work concepts, the values of the program will almost certainly shift from those core concepts to reflect a more task oriented, accountability-based approach to the work.
- The onus is always on the supervisor to explore whether what child and youth workers say they do is what they actually do. Just because a child and youth worker claims to be engaging the clients does not mean that there actually is any engagement going on. Supervisors have to ensure that language does not become a substitute for performance.
- Since so much of child and youth work unfolds in a team context, the target of performance management cannot be limited to individual workers. The team itself must also be subject to the process of performance management. There are many excellent child and youth workers who became quite dysfunctional within the context of their team (Fulcher, 2007; Kruger, 1987).
- Finally, and perhaps most importantly, the most significant but also most complex source of information for understanding the performance of a child and youth worker are, of course, the clients. Ultimately, the work of a child and youth worker is measured against how a client is experiencing that work, and only the client can effectively speak to this. For this reason, it is always imperative that a manager or supervisor maintain an ongoing dialogue with the clients that can serve to ascertain how they might be experiencing the work of the child and youth workers involved with them without placing the burden of performance management on them.

Performance management entails a great deal more; however, these few points capture some of the things that might not be included in the training delivered by HR specialists or administrators. It is always critical to remember that a child and youth work environment is a unique one indeed, and therefore every process that unfolds must in some way take account of the unique aspects of our profession. As previously indicated, one of the core processes of performance management in child and youth care practice is the process of supervision. Supervision is, however, much more than just about performance management. It also contributes to quality assurance, individual and team morale, self care for workers, and sometimes even clinical intervention in worker-client relationships. Given the importance of supervision in virtually every aspect of child and youth care practice, we will explore this process in greater detail below, and we will suggest some of the themes that might be explored during supervision sessions as well.

SUPERVISION STANDARDS IN CHILD AND YOUTH CARE PRACTICE

Supervision has long been recognized as a core component of many human services professions, including social work (Cearley, 2004). Much of the literature on supervision within the child and youth care field focuses on three major points (Delano, 2001; Garfat, 2001; Magnuson & Burger, 2001; Maier, 1985; Mann-Feder, 2001; Phelan, 1990; Ricks, 1989):

- Supervision is essential in order for a child and youth worker to be able to effectively do the job.
- Supervision is a long term process that includes both supervision sessions and exploration and dialogue between these sessions.
- Supervision is distinct from teaching, training, and redirection, and is instead better understood as a process of exploration that a supervisor and supervisee are engaged in jointly.

Supervision is arguably one of the most challenging parts of being a manager. This is because as a manager, we tend to want things to always be better than they currently are, but we are not in fact in control of how things are at any given time. Moreover, supervisors are placed in supervisory positions for all kinds of reasons, but almost never because higher managers in the agency or administrators believe them to be excellent supervisors. More commonly, the reasons for promotion are based on administrative excellence, demonstrated excellence in front line duties, or educational qualifications. Most new supervisors would typically never have had the opportunity to try out their supervision skills before becoming a supervisor. The only major exception to this is where a front line child and youth worker has the opportunity to supervise a placement student. However, one of the major differences between supervising a placement student versus supervising an employee is that in the case of the former, teaching, guidance, and redirection are in fact major components of the supervision process.

A meaningful way to get started in the provision of supervision is to reflect on what the purpose of this process really is. We could identify a number of possible purposes (Gilbert & Charles, 2001; Seibel, 2001):

- It is an opportunity for the supervisor to find out what is actually happening in the program.
- It is an opportunity for the child and youth worker to speak honestly and directly to his or her perspective on what is actually happening in the program.
- It is an opportunity to reflect on and perhaps problem solve around specific issues that may exist with respect to team dynamics, particular clients, or other program-related issues.
- It is an opportunity for the child and youth worker to step back from the day-to-day turmoil of the work and reflect with the supervisor on the *meaning* of the work.
- Related to the above, it is an opportunity to compare what we do with the core concepts of child and youth work at a more abstract level.

It is probably fair to say that child and youth workers are subject to a great deal of unpredicted input in their day-to-day activities. Under these circumstances, it is very easy to lose sight of any particular way of thinking, or any particular frame of reference that brings together practical strategies for *doing* child and youth work with more value-based and theoretical thinking about *being* a child and youth worker. Without a doubt, one of the major goals of supervision is to ensure that these all important processes of self-reflection, critical thinking, and exploration of the values that guide our work do not get lost.

Having said this, frequently the agenda of a supervisor (particularly a good one) does not exactly correspond to the agenda of the child and youth worker. The latter often wants solutions, concrete advice, and a discussion that focuses on his day-to-day reality. The supervisor, in contrast, wants to ensure that the child and youth worker has an opportunity to step back from that day-to-day reality, think in less concrete terms and takes the time to reflect on *meaning* as much as he reflects on *action*.

This means that the supervision process has to find a way of incorporating both agendas. This is not always easy, and there certainly is no sure fire way of doing so or no template that can achieve this in every case. Nevertheless, there are a number of themes and discussion topics that might serve to tie together practical issues with reflective opportunities:

Theme 1: Relationship-building with Youth

Possible discussion topics:

1. What steps have you taken to build a meaningful relationship with any of the children/youth in the program (family, classroom, unit) during the past month?
2. How do you reflect on your identity as you build this relationship?
3. How do you reflect on and incorporate the identity of the child or youth in the context of family, community and other life spaces?
4. What have you brought to the children/youth that may be experienced as rewarding, nurturing, or helpful?
5. What barriers have you faced in your attempts to build a relationship with each of the children/youth in the program (each member of the family in the case of in-home support programs; each student in the case of school-based programs)?

Theme 2: Active Engagement

Possible discussion topics:

1. What have you done to actively engage each of the children/youth (or family members) during the past month?
2. What activities have you planned and followed through on?
3. How much time are you spending in the office (or doing administrative work) and for what reasons are you there?
4. What has each of the children/youth been thinking about during the past month, and how have you assisted them in working through those thoughts?

Theme 3: Compliance

Possible discussion topics:

1. How have you assisted the children/youth in reflecting on issues of noncompliance with the expectations of the program?
2. Where and when have you imposed expectations that reflect your needs versus the needs of the children/youth?
3. What consequences have you imposed during the past month (or have you recommended be imposed within the context of family-based settings) and how do these relate to the unique needs of the children/youth involved?
4. In what kinds of situations have you considered the specific needs of a child/youth to come before the requirements of the program, and what was your reasoning?

Theme 4: Caring/Nurture

Possible discussion topics:

1. What are some examples of nurture that you implemented during the past month?
2. What other approaches to nurture might you have considered?
3. Where do you see a need to increase nurture with a particular child/youth and how do you propose we do so?
4. What nurturing have you seen unfold at the hands of your colleagues (in team-based settings; family members in in-home support programs) during the past month?

Theme 5: Accountability

Possible discussion topics:

1. What accountability measures have you imposed during the past month?
2. How have specific children/youth experienced these accountability measures?
3. What steps have you taken that you yourself remain accountable in terms of having provided nurturing and meaningful service to the children/youth in the program?

4. What follow up steps have you taken in order to ensure that your accountability measures remain meaningful beyond the moment of imposition?

Theme 6: Communication

Possible discussion topics:

1. How often have you spoken to another professional outside of our program during the past month?
2. What steps have you taken in order to ensure that your colleagues are aware of your specific perspective on the child/youth?
3. What advocacy on behalf of the child/youth have you been involved with during this past month?
4. What other community services have you communicated with during this past month?
5. Have you had contact with the neighbors, peers or other important persons in the life of the child or youth?

Additional Themes to Explore:

1. What are your plans for the coming month?
2. What special interaction are you planning with what child/youth and how does this further your relationship with the child/youth?
3. How will you support your colleagues during the coming month?
4. What are your agenda items for the next team meeting?
5. Review the Plan of Care (if applicable) for any of your assigned children or youth.

Each program and each scenario has its own unique features that may require additions or deletions to this particular set of themes and discussion topics. In a different context, one might want to adjust the themes and discussion topics somewhat to reflect on other areas of activity. Where one is dealing with a team of child and youth workers where most have pre-service qualifications that include a Child and Youth Worker Diploma or Degree, another theme around the core concept of Self-Reflection might be appropriate and viable (Mann-Feder, 2001).

Of course, supervision is an entirely different proposition when we, as child and youth workers in a supervisory position, supervise professionals from other disciplines. It is worthwhile to briefly consider this issue as well.

Supervising Professionals from Other Disciplines

The first thing we can say about this particular scenario is that it does not happen very often. If we think about the kinds of professions that might be involved in the programs we could potentially manage, many are such that their supervision tends to either be non-existent, or alternatively take place in an entirely different context. Thus, professionals like doctors, psychiatrists, and psychologists, as well as nurses, either are supervised by regulatory systems such as the College of Physicians or they simply do not receive nor want to receive any sort of supervision. One of the obvious problems from our perspective is that we generally lack the expertise related to their specific work focus anyway (although this has never stopped other professions from supervising us!). And yet it is exactly in relation to their involvement that child and youth workers often encounter some tension. How often have we heard child and youth workers complain about the unilateral decision-making of a psychiatrist based on only very brief contact with a child or youth, or the go-it-alone attitude of a nurse when developing a nutritional plan for a particular youth?

As a manager, we are the person in charge of the program, and we cannot simply abdicate our responsibility toward certain aspects of the program because we cannot effectively supervise particular professions. This means that we have to adjust the supervision process to reflect our relationship with these professions and to target the role of those professions within our programs (Keliher, 2005; Salhani & Charles, 2007). By role, I mean at least two things:

- How does a particular professional impact the clients?
- How does the professional impact the child and youth workers and their day-to-day work?

With respect to the first question, the purpose of supervision might be more accurately articulated as being to ensure that any profession involved with the program and specific clients complements the work of the child and youth care team as opposed to taking place along side of it. If indeed a particular service is to be part of the program, we are responsible for ensuring that this service is integrated into the overall service provided by the program, and therefore corresponds to the program's goals and objectives. We do not have to know much about the content of the work of a psychiatrist in order to judge whether that work is unfolding in an integrated manner or a disjointed and *ad hoc* manner.

With respect to the second question, we are back to a uniquely child and youth work way of seeing the world. Our specific concern here is not so much about the content of a particular function served by other professionals, but instead we are concerned with how that function is being experienced by others, notably our child and youth workers. In the end, we remain committed to the idea that what actually happens is always secondary to how those impacted make meaning of what happens.

A great deal of the challenge of supervising other professions mirrors some of the challenges entailed in what is almost always the case when child and youth workers become managers. Sure, we are given added responsibilities and considerable authority over *some things*; yet, in the vast majority of situations, child and youth workers become middle managers at best. This renders us vulnerable to the many traps of middle management.

Middle Management Traps

As middle managers, we still have a boss, and usually several bosses. And those bosses are almost never child and youth workers. This has all kinds of implications. First, the higher up the ladder of management, the more significant corporate considerations figure in thinking. While service managers might want to talk to the boss about service related things, the boss will likely hear them through the filter of corporate considerations, including costs, HR implications, and public relations issues. Also very high on the boss's agenda will be the issue of risk management, which is a very annoying topic for child and youth workers who always work within the context of at best scantily managed risk.

Perhaps the greatest challenge will be to manage the often conflicting directions of those who are supervised by the middle manager versus those who give him direction. While the middle manager is busy trying to keep the child and youth workers motivated, direction may be given by upper management that directly conflicts with the goals and aspirations of the child and youth workers. For example, while the child and youth care practitioner in a middle management position might want to take an approach to performance management with a particular child and youth worker that reflects some of the profession's unique features, as discussed earlier, the senior manager may impose an HR approach instead, resulting in the middle manager having to do something that to the child and youth workers will undoubtedly appear as hypocritical.

Typically, if a middle manager is unable to assert himself with the higher levels of management, he runs the risk of being viewed as not overly relevant by the child and youth workers. Rather than paying attention to him, they will wait and see what the real bosses have to say. If, on the other hand, the middle manager comes on too strongly in trying to assert himself amongst the higher levels of management, then either his own management career may come to an unexpected end, or he will find himself passed over when interesting projects or opportunities come up.

It is possible to mitigate some of the implications of the middle management trap, but this will require a significant focus on language and communication. Child and youth work language is not going to make a great deal of sense to an HR specialist or the chief financial officer of the agency, or even some of the service directors within the agency. In the context of a school board or a hospital for example, the area of responsibility of the middle manager is almost certainly at best a minor part of the bureaucracy's operation. All bureaucracies will protect the core of their operations over the add-ons, and therefore the middle manager will have to somehow make sure to always use language that clearly connects the significance of his operation to the well being of the core operation of the bureaucracy. There are several ways in which this can be done:

- Developing partnerships and joint initiatives with other departments within the agency;
- Awareness of and fluency in the language of other departments (for example, HR language, financial language, clinical language, quality assurance language);
- Framing activities and initiatives within the legislative and regulatory contexts of the broader organization's mandate.

As child and youth workers, we have learned to focus on the children, youth and families we are involved with, to live through their experiences, to be engaged and to have or be in relationships. Management positions represent somewhat of a challenge to the integrity of child and youth care intentions. Management is the domain of the pragmatist. As child and youth care practitioners in management positions, we should never compromise our values and beliefs, and we should always advocate for the ideals of our profession. But we cannot be entirely dogmatic about this. Much like we know that we cannot simply tell our clients to get better, to grow, and to learn, other professionals, administrators, and bureaucracies cannot be told to accept our values and beliefs; they will have to experience their benefits and everybody and every entity experiences things only on their terms.

BARRIERS FOR EFFECTIVE CHILD AND YOUTH CARE MANAGERS

Most child and youth workers are not quite ready to become managers, but that is true for most professionals from all disciplines ascending to the ranks of management for the first time. Therefore, a lack of readiness is not necessarily a problem. It does, however, necessitate that new managers quickly and honestly develop a list of skills and resources that may need to be acquired as soon as possible. Several of these are discussed below.

Program Evaluation Skills

While working directly with children, youth or families, child and youth care practitioners are not typically too concerned about whether what they are doing is efficient, effective and sustainable. This may sound strange, since surely all child and youth care practitioners would like to do the best job possible, but it reflects a focus on the "day to day doing" versus a focus on a more systematic approach to evaluating the outcomes of what is being done. As a manager, it becomes necessary to have at least some basic skills in program evaluation approaches. Perhaps even more minimally, a manager needs to know what program evaluation really is, and how to get started in the process even if one were to contract this particular task out to someone with greater expertise in this process. The importance of program evaluation transcends the desire to provide the best possible service to clients; it also serves the purpose of ensuring that the manager can meaningfully discuss the program with other managers in the organization, and can back up requests for resources with actual data related to program outcomes. Without understanding at least the basics of program evaluation, a manager's representation of the program is essentially entirely anecdotal, which creates significant limitations in terms of credibility and possibilities for program expansion through added resources (Merton, Comfort, & Payne, 2007; Subhra, 2007).

Research and Literature

Very much related to the issue of program evaluation is the issue of research and literature relevant to the services being managed. It is important for a manager to be able to situate the program's structure and activities within a body of research and literature (Furstenau, 2000). Particularly given the current enthusiasm for evidence-based practice, the knowledge about current research findings related to the type of program one is responsible for is invaluable. This requires that managers maintain themselves up to date in terms of where to find such research reports and how to read and understand them. The field of child and youth care is increasingly producing large numbers of research-based reports and studies that are immediately relevant to practitioners and managers in service environments. While this is indeed a positive development in our field, it is only useful if all of this research is actually accessed by those who could use the findings to improve their own programs or develop new ones. An awareness of the major academic journals in the field as well as institutions and organization producing research-based reports on a regular basis is therefore indispensable.

Not everything that is published in the field is research-based, at least not in the sense that it reflects outcome findings or evidence bases of particular approaches to service provision. A great deal of literature is theoretical or conceptual, but this too is useful in order to frame one's activities as a manager within a well-thought out and publicly discussed conceptual frame. The ability to point to academic or professional leaders' work as a reference point for specific decisions or management approaches adds credibility and likely will elicit much more support and enthusiasm from senior managers or funders.

Time Management

An immediate challenge facing managers in the field of child and youth care is time management, arguably one of the most critical skills required for management in any profession. As front line workers, time management for child and youth workers is largely reflective of the activities of clients and the demands of particular program designs. Particularly for child and youth workers in nonresidential settings, time management can still be a significant issue, since the time demands of clients cannot be managed within the structured framework of a specific program that has similar expectations of all the clients. Child and youth workers working with families in their homes, for example, may encounter family demands that vary considerably from family to family, and this can result in significant time management challenges. Nevertheless, even in such cases, the pressure to manage time is very much related to our obligations towards clients, and only minimally to our obligations toward the agency, colleagues or the community at large.

As managers, child and youth workers quickly realize that time management is an entirely different concept, driven less by the demands or needs of clients, and more by the virtually limitless needs of adults. Adults include those for whom the manager is responsible as a supervisor, but also families who may have concerns about a service, other managers in the agency, other professionals from other disciplines both within and outside of the agency, neighbors, community members, partner organizations, consultants, regulators and a host of others. One of the challenges associated with managing all of these adult relationships is that while each relationship is one of many for the manager, for the adult concerned the manager is the central figure in whatever the issue, concern or task at hand might be. Every request and every task is typically framed as a priority by the other party, and it is impossible for the manager to respond to all of these as priorities. Ultimately, effective time management in a child and youth care context requires that the manager develop some basic principles against which all requests and concerns are measured in terms of their priority status. As we will explore further below, one such principle surely will reflect the everyday need to care for children and youth in the program and to do so in accordance with the best and most sophisticated practical and conceptual tools the discipline of child and youth care has to offer.

Loyalty and Boundary Issues

Adult relationships are indeed far more complex and time consuming than the relationships we develop with children or youth, and in some cases, such relationships can really challenge managers in a child and youth care context. Particularly for new managers or supervisors who were appointed to the position directly from the team they now supervise, adult relationships are supremely challenging. In a best-case scenario, the new manager is accepted by the team as the best choice for the position, and team members will maintain an open mind and a supportive stance toward the new manager. More commonly, however, there is not typically such a consensus amongst team members, and while some may well be supportive, others undoubtedly will harbor less positive feelings about the new manager having achieved a position of authority and prestige when they have not.

Perhaps even more complicated are situations where new managers are placed in a position where they have to supervise their former friends. Friendships and sometimes more intimate relationships are very common particularly in residential child and youth care settings, and it is not atypical for newly appointed supervisors to have somewhat of a history amongst their team members. For the new manager, managing longstanding relationships that now have a hierarchical basis is extremely challenging, and doing so in a way that is accepted not only by the parties to such relationships but also by those members of the team who did not have particularly strong relationships with the new manager is even more challenging and sometimes not possible. Without a doubt, these scenarios require extraordinarily strong skills in terms of boundary development and articulating rationales for such boundaries on the part of the new manager.

One of the costs of becoming a manager in an agency where one has previously worked front line is therefore related to changes in relationships that may have had strong personal components. Maintaining such relationships long term and trying to separate one's professional and personal interaction with a child and youth worker is almost never a good plan. This is one of the reasons why child and youth workers with management aspirations are well advised to seek out management positions in other agencies wherever possible, or at least in other departments of the same agency where possible.

Finding Peers

Management positions in child and youth care environments can be lonely at times; this is because in most agencies, management personnel have quite disparate responsibilities and are concerned about different kinds of issues. Although the job is without a doubt a very busy one, and one that involves a great deal of adult and client interaction, many child and youth care managers find themselves alone in their day-to-day responsibilities and the issues they face while fulfilling these responsibilities. It does not help that child and youth care practitioners typically have very close knit relationships with their colleagues and rely on their colleagues for constructive feedback as well as for venting and de-briefing purposes. Once a child and youth care practitioner assumes a management position, these support systems are gone. It is generally quite inappropriate and perhaps even unprofessional to vent one's "management frustrations" to those one is supervising. At the same time, many management colleagues may or may not be able to relate to the kinds of issues commonly facing the child and youth care manager.

This is why it is important, wherever possible, to develop a new professional peer group that may have to extend beyond the reach of one's own agency. While most agencies operate only one residential program, one education program or one family support program, each agency has a manager for such a program, and these are the people who a newly appointed child and youth care manager ought to be seeking out. Support can come in many forms and shape, but support from individuals with similar responsibilities and concerns is essential to maintain a healthy and effective outlook on one's job. After all, this is one of the core advantages of working in a team when working front line, and similarly, it generates a great deal of advantage when working solo as a manager in an agency where there is only one child and youth care manager.

Unions

One of the major changes experienced by managers who have moved from the front lines to the ranks of management is the new relationship that must be developed with the union in those workplaces that are unionized. While there are not too many such workplaces in some jurisdictions (such as the United States), there are increasingly many in others (such as in Canada and in many European countries). Unions are complex institutions that have tremendous impact on the employment context of child and youth workers. In some organizations, employer–employee relationships are relatively smooth, giving the appearance of minimal union impact. In others, these relationships are tense and there are constant power struggles between the union and the employer.

As a child and youth worker in a management position, it is enormously difficult to maintain a child and youth work approach to managing performance when one is also dealing with an aggressive and combatant union. One of the common issues in this relationship is that unions often represent child and youth workers only by default; their main reason for being is to represent other disciplines, often social workers or teachers. As a result, union executives frequently know very little about the nuances of child and youth care, and maintain the same positions with respect to employment issues that arise for child and youth workers as they do in other circumstances.

As a manager, the requirements of collective agreements struck with unions can often be quite challenging to implement. In a residential context, for example, health and safety regulations enshrined in the collective agreement may prohibit child and youth workers from changing a light bulb if this requires the use of a ladder; appropriately trained maintenance workers must do so instead, but this might leave the residents (and staff) in the dark for days until such a maintenance person is available to do the job. Call-in procedures for emergency staffing may not allow a supervisor to consider the best possible match for a particular client in need of extra support, and instead dogmatically insist on seniority as the criteria for who is offered the shift.

In nonresidential contexts, other impediments to doing child and youth care may be in place. In some organizations, the collective agreements have provisions whereby workers can refuse to enter the homes of clients who smoke; this is surely a difficult obstacle to child and youth workers seeking to establish a relationship with a family. Similarly, requirements related to hours of work can render it prohibitive for a child and youth worker to see a family in crisis after already having completed an eight hour work day, since this would then be overtime that may have to be offered to someone else based on seniority.

While unions are primarily concerned about due process, child and youth care managers must find ways of implementing programs that by their very nature require a high degree of pragmatism and flexibility, particularly in nonresidential settings. Negotiating exceptions with a union can be very difficult, since such exceptions are always precedent setting and therefore can become major obstacles from the perspective of union executives. On the other hand, failing to engage with the union means capitulating to processes and procedures that may well be detrimental to children and youth, and that surely is not an option.

Perhaps the greatest frustration around dealing with union issues relates to the inability of the child and youth care manager in a middle management position to make final decisions about specific situations. Since union–employer relationships are managed at the highest level of both the union and the employer, child and youth care managers are frequently only the first step in a grievance process, and their decisions about the situation will have to be vetted through the human resource machinery of the agency before it can stand.

All of the issues explored above are *potential* barriers to effective management approaches for child and youth care practitioners. This means that there typically are ways of mitigating the impacts of these barriers, and ensuring that the job of the child and youth care manager can in fact be done effectively and without resulting in the quick burnout of the manager. In order to ensure that the job remains viable and maintains its opportunities for positively impacting on the services provided to children, youth and families, child and youth care practitioners in management positions need to articulate a professional identity for themselves. This is what we will explore as the final element of this article on child and youth care approaches to management.

A PROFESSIONAL IDENTITY FOR CHILD AND YOUTH CARE MANAGERS

Child and youth care practitioners who enter the field of management are at a constant risk of losing their professional identity. As we have seen above, the pressures of management positions are such that the norms and procedures of other disciplines, such as human resource management, quickly take over and become the *modus operandi* of the day-to-day work. From an agency perspective, managers, and especially middle managers, are there to solve problems, and typically the most efficient approach is also deemed the most desirable.

In this way, the basic principles of the child and youth care profession are not inherently compatible with the operational logic of management. Particularly the focus on process that is critical in child and youth care practice is difficult to reconcile with the need to produce sustainable outcomes that limit the risk exposure of the agency and eliminate chronic problems, including chronically weak or ineffective staff. Ignoring the expectations of agency management customs in favor of maintaining an approach that is firmly rooted in child and youth care principles is not an effective strategy for the child and youth care manager. Managers too are subject to performance management, and the management career of the child and youth care practitioners will come to an abrupt halt if indeed the agency's expectations are not met. A more effective approach, therefore, involves a great deal of pragmatism, but never to the degree of sacrificing the professional ethics and norms of the child and youth care profession altogether. In order to develop a framework for action, the child and youth care manager needs to develop a professional identity that speaks both to the principles of child and youth care as a profession and to the requirements and expectations of management procedures.

Any professional identity must be based on a set of principles that has philosophical merit and operational value. Child and youth care practice has based its professional identity on a series of concepts that remain central to working in the profession. These include the concepts of boundaries, relationships, engagement and being with clients in their life spaces. Regardless of the specific employment context and the particular policies and procedures in place within any given agency, child and youth care practitioners seek to give life and meaning to these central concepts, adjusting operationally to the employment context but philosophically remaining committed to the approach derived from the interdependencies of these concepts. Similarly, the child and youth care manager can identify a series of concepts that can help to remain centered within the child and youth care profession but that can also extend to interdependencies with management concepts and procedures. Based on our discussions above, we can readily identify four such concepts: a focus on process along with outcomes, resilience building, decision-making and maintaining an uncompromising commitment to the preservation of children's rights and the ethics of the profession.

The Value of Process

In a relational profession, the role of process cannot possibly be overstated. Virtually everything we do as child and youth care practitioners is based on our belief that the process of doing so itself provides opportunities for meaning making and personal growth. Change is seen as an inevitable by-product of process, and therefore a well thought out process gives rise to positive change over time. With this principle in hand, the child and youth care manager must commit to process as much as to the achievement of outcomes. Perhaps most critically, allowing process to drive performance management procedures will ensure that child and youth care practitioners experience their interactions with the manager within a framework that is consistent with their own day-to-day activities and therefore familiar to them.

Change is a major challenge in virtually all work environments, and perhaps even more so in child and youth care environments. One reason for this is that change at any level in such an environment impacts on all levels of that environment. Trying to generate greater efficiency in a staffing schedule, for example, is not only about persuading the staff to work at different times or different kinds of shifts, but it is also about managing the experience children and youth will have under the new schedule. It is therefore not advisable to do what managers in other disciplines, and particularly in the administrative disciplines, do all too often: pushing change at a pace that exceeds a system's capacity to absorb change. Child and youth care managers should always maintain this most basic of child and youth care principles: Process *is* change, and the benefits of change are entirely dependent on the capacity to absorb change, which will almost certainly vary considerably from person to person, staff to staff and client to client. The concept of life space also becomes relevant in this context. The wise child and youth care manager will always remember that a change to any aspect of a program, whether it is targeting the human resources of that program, the financial structures of the program or even the physical appearance of that program, constitutes a change in the life space of the child. It is therefore never appropriate to make such changes without due consideration to time frames that are meaningful to those involved in this life space, procedures that are understandable and rationales that make sense from a child and youth care perspective.

One core element of the professional identity of the child and youth care manager, therefore, is the commitment to process as the core element of the management approach.

Resilience Builders

Whereas most management theory is focused on the elimination of problems and pursuing an ideal state of operational functioning, child and youth care approaches to management are based on the core principles of resilience theory. As a child and youth care manager, it is important to accept that staffing resources much like clients will continuously encounter challenges and adversity in their day-to-day lives and activities. Moreover, given the unpredictable nature of the life spaces in which child and youth care unfolds, whether in a residential context, in schools, in hospitals or in the community, the idea that one can eliminate problems and create procedural environments that meaningfully limit risk exposure and conflict is unrealistic. Instead, child and youth care managers focus on what child and youth care practitioners focus on with respect to children and youth: they seek to build resilience amongst their staff, within their programs and amongst their clients so that the unexpected challenges and problems can be absorbed into the day-to-day experience of the program and all of its components without derailing the program altogether.

Building resilience requires a focus on the well-being of staff, both in their professional lives and in their private lives to the extent that these are accessible to the manager. It requires giving a voice to staff and clients alike in how the program is structured and how it operates, and it requires responding quickly and meaningfully to concerns or discomforts cited by staff or clients. Resilience research has demonstrated effectively that the ability to overcome adversity is a function of both internal and external capacities and resources; the effective child and youth care manager will seek to contribute to maintaining the highest possible standards with respect to these capacities and resources, and he will work hard to provide whatever supports are needed to continuously strengthen these resilience building factors.

Decision-makers

Notwithstanding the incorporation of process and resilience building as core elements of the professional identity of the child and youth care manager, the concept of decision-making is also central in effective management approaches. Certainly it is within the framework of decision-making that the child and youth care manager will be evaluated by the senior managers of an agency. Outcomes are always linked to decisions, and as middle managers, in spite of the limitations imposed by broader organizational considerations, decision-making is a daily task. In and of itself, decision-making does not violate the principles of process and resilience building, but it is within the context of decision-making that these principles are at greatest risk. Decisions that appear random, heavy handed or uncompromising will not be easily reconciled with the commitment to process, and decisions that may add responsibilities or expectations to staff will not easily be seen as contributing to their resilience.

On the other hand, child and youth care practitioners as well as children and youth already experience a great deal of uncertainty in their lives, and the absence of decision-making on the part of the manager may contribute further to these experiences. There are, therefore, times when everyone looks to the leader to make a decision for no other reason than to move forward and to create an opportunity for everyone to commit to a specific direction or approach. Particularly in a team context, the need to provide direction for the whole team is often necessary in order to break through situations where an excess of differing opinions or approaches is causing chaos or disarray.

The core element of effective decision-making is not typically the decision itself but rather the rationale associated with that decision. A child and youth care manager cannot abdicate the responsibility to make decisions, but he can certainly work hard to ensure that the rationale for decisions is well framed within the research evidence and the conceptual literature of child and youth care. The opportunities for action borne out of any given decision still provide flexibility to accommodate the particular strengths and competencies of all staff members and clients.

Children's Rights and Ethics

The purpose of having a professional identity in any profession is to be able to frame one's actions within some core principles of identity.

Ultimately, the child and youth care manager must be able to answer (for himself and for others) this question: *What do you stand for?* While we often affirm our position that there are no right or wrong answers in our profession, this simple question in an exception. There is in fact a right answer to this question: *I stand for the protection of children's rights and the preservation of ethical standards in all activities which I have the privilege to lead!* The child and youth care manager can acknowledge that there may well be myriad ways of achieving these goals, however, the goals themselves are not flexible. Therefore, as part of the professional identity of the child and youth care manager, it ought to be known to everyone—including the children and youth in the program, the staff, and the management team of the agency—that the manager will always act in accordance with a sophisticated understanding of children's rights and ethical conduct, defined by the Code of Ethics of the child and youth care profession.

The importance of this element of the professional identity of the child and youth care manager is not always obvious, particularly at a very practical level. And yet it is this element that will serve to make the management approach of the child and youth care manager effective and transparent. In a residential setting, for example, staff may want to use food as a consequence for bad behavior. The manager's response will be to disallow this not because of loyalty to those arguing against it and not because of personal preferences about how to consequence children for their negative behaviors, but simply because children have a right to healthy, nutritious food that reflects their cultural and religious traditions, and therefore there is no room for using food as a consequence. Once child and youth care practitioners begin to understand that children's rights are paramount in the decision-making of the manager, requests for policies or procedures that limit or violate those rights will disappear or at least decrease in frequency. In a school setting, the staff might want to use an isolation room as a way of controlling the behavior of a specific child. Again, the manager will disallow this simply because children have a right to education, and this right will be violated if the child spends excessive periods of time in the isolation room.

The focus on ethics will also provide clarity in terms of responding to requests from senior management. For example, during difficult financial times, the child and youth care manager might well be asked to eliminate professional development activities due to costs. The response, in accordance with the ethical requirement to maintain up to date with current best practices in the field, will surely be that such activities cannot be eliminated as per ethical requirements. And still, there might be opportunities for providing such professional development activities in ways that are more cost effective and efficient, and therefore can meet both the requests of senior managers and the ethical standards of the profession. Finding these ways is what the job of the manager is all about. Knowing the parameters within which to make decisions about what the priorities are, what can be eliminated temporarily and what must absolutely remain in place reflects a strong sense of professional identity on the part of the child and youth care manager.

Management in child and youth care contexts is a difficult task that will challenge the professional integrity of the child and youth care practitioner. The demands of the job are high, the resources are usually limited, and the scenarios that might become relevant are virtually unlimited. On the other hand, these are the kinds of positions that will provide opportunities for child and youth care practitioners to exercise leadership in the ongoing development of the profession, and to ensure that the development of the profession proceeds with the principles of child and youth care practice protected and nurtured. While the professional issues for child and youth workers that are associated with taking on management responsibilities are endless, the poor representation of the profession at management levels in agencies and organizations across the social service sectors itself constitutes a major professional issue for the discipline of child and youth care. We have come a long way from our humble beginnings in highly institutionalized residential care; the time to move in all directions, including up, is now.

REFERENCES

Bracey, M. (2007). The accidental leader. In R. Harrison, C. Benjamin, S. Curran, & R. Hunter (Eds.), *Leading work with young people* (pp. 25–33). London: SAGE.

Cearley, S. (2004). The power of supervision in child welfare services. *Child and Youth Care Forum, 33*(5), 313–327.

Delano, F. (2001). If I could supervise my supervisor: A model for child and youth care workers to "own their own supervision." *Journal of Child and Youth Care, 15*(2), 51–64.

Ferguson, R. (1982). The role of university child care training programs in the development of a professional career ladder for child care workers. *Journal of Child and Youth Care, 1*(1), 67–70.

Flint, B. M. (1966). *The child and the institution: A study of deprivation and recovery.* Toronto, Canada: University of Toronto Press.

Fulcher, L. C. (2007). Residential child and youth care is fundamentally about team work. *Relational Child and Youth Care Practice, 20*(4), 30–36.

Furstenau, P. (2000). The role of research skills in the curriculum for child & youth care. *Journal of Child and Youth Care, 14*(1), 49–54.

Garfat, T. (2001). Congruence between supervision and practice. *Journal of Child and Youth Care. 15*(2), iii–iv.

Gharabaghi, K. (2005). Our greatest failure. *Relational Child and Youth Care Practice, 18*(3), 60–61.

Gilbert, S., & Charles, G. (2001). Great child and youth care practice: The foundation for great supervision. *Journal of Child and Youth Care, 15*(2), 23–32.

Harrison, R., Benjamin, C., Curran, S., & Hunter, R. (2007). Introduction. In R. Harrison, C. Benjamin, S. Curran, & R. Hunter (Eds.), *Leading work with young people* (pp. 1–3). London: SAGE.

Ingram, G., & Harris, J. (2001). *Delivering good youth work: A working guide to thriving and surviving.* Dorset, UK: Russell House Publishing.

Kay, H., Kendrick, A., Davidson, J., & Stevens, I. (2007). Safer recruitment: Protecting children, improving practice in residential child care. *Child Abuse Review, 16*(4), 223–226.

Keliher, M. N. (2005). In defense of the interdisciplinary team and the role of the child and youth care worker. *Relational Child and Youth Care Practice, 18*(3), 63–68.

Klopovic, J., Vasu, M. L., & Yearwood, D. L. (2003). *Effective program practices for at-risk youth: A continuum of community-based programs.* Kingston, NJ: Civic Research Institute.

Krueger, M. (1986). Making the team approach work in residential group care. *Child Welfare, 66*, 447–57.

Linton, T. E., & Fox, L. (1986). The child and youth care worker: Marginal employee or professional team member? *Residential Group Care and Treatment, 3*(4), 39–54.

Magnuson, D., & Burger, L. (2001). Developmental supervision in residential care. *Journal of Child and Youth Care, 15*(1), 9–22.

Maier, H. W. (1985). Teaching and training as a facet of supervision of child care staff: An overview. *Journal of Child Care, 2*(4), 49–52.

Mann-Feder, V. (2001). The self as subject in child and youth care supervision. *Journal of Child and Youth Care, 15*(2), 1–8.

Merton, B., Comfort, H., & Payne, M. (2007). Recognizing and recording the impact of youth work. In R. Harrison, C. Benjamin, S. Curran, & R. Hunter (Eds.), *Leading work with young people* (pp. 271–284). London: SAGE.

Phelan, J. (1990). Child care supervision: The neglected skill of evaluation. In J. P. Anglin, C. J. Denhom, R. V. Ferfuson, & A. R. Pence (Eds.), *Perspectives in professional child and youth care* (pp. 127–141). New York: Haworth.

Ricks, F. (1989). Self-awareness model for training and application in child and youth care. *Journal of Child and Youth Care, 4*(1), 33–41.

Salhani, D., & Charles, G. (2007). The dynamics of an inter-professional team: The interplay of child and youth care with other professions within a residential treatment milieu. *Relational Child and Youth Care Practice, 20*(4), 12–20.

Seibel, D. K. (2001). Fire setting, fire fighting or fire prevention: Understanding and succeeding at the complex role of supervisor in child and youth care. *Journal of Child and Youth Care, 15*(2), 73–82.

Stuart, C., & Sanders, L. (2008). *Child and youth care practitioners' contributions to evidence-based practice in group care.* Toronto, Canada: Ryerson University.

Subhra, G. (2007). Reclaiming the evaluation agenda. In R. Harrison, C. Benjamin, S. Curran, & R. Hunter (Eds.), *Leading work with young people* (pp. 285–298). London: SAGE.

VanderVen, K. (1998). View from the field: Holding out for higher education. *Journal of Child and Youth Care, 12*(4), 95–98.

Warner, N. (1992). *Choosing with care: The report of the committee of inquiry into the selection, development and management of staff in children's homes.* London: HMSO.

CONCLUSION: WHERE TO FROM HERE?

Writing about professional issues in child and youth care practice is a little bit like extracting the salt from the oceans' waters. In that process, we are not really removing the salt as a distinct substance, but instead we remove the water and deem whatever is left behind as 'sea salt'. Similarly, we can never be quite sure whether what we are discussing or exploring in our field is indeed a professional issue as opposed to any other kind of issue. In practice, child and youth care comes as a package in which we, as professionals, are part and parcel of the services we provide. It is therefore very important that practitioners remain conscious of the ambiguities entailed in relation to the professional issues in our discipline. Much of what has been explored in this book is meant to provide a framework for evaluating one's practice critically, and perhaps even for advancing the profession itself by raising the standards related to language and articulation as well as the depth of understanding of what we do, day in and day out, in the life space(s) of children, youth and their families.

It is nevertheless possible to summarize the main themes explored in this book by focusing on four issues in particular. Together, these four issues represent the foundation for not only strong practice, but also for ensuring that practitioners are viewed and see themselves as a larger project and a meaningful professional discipline. The four issues are: professional identity, professional conduct, professional competence and a deep commitment to being with young people in a democratic manner. It is notable that these issues mirror many of the messages articulated by some of the core contributors to our discipline from the past and into the present (Bettelheim, 1974; Brendtro, Brokenleg & VanB, 1990; Brendtro, Ness & Mitchell, 2005; Redl & Wineman, 1952). Professional issues in child and youth care practice may have expanded as a result of the increasing complexities of service systems and the much increased deployment of practitioners in myriad service settings, but the core nature of these issues has by and large remained the same. By way of ensuring the message of this book has been delivered, each of these issues will be explored one more time to conclude this book.

PROFESSIONAL IDENTITY

The historical marginalization of those directly involved with young people on a day to day basis in care-giving roles has been very unhelpful in terms of developing a strong professional identity for the discipline. It has, however, been quite impactful in terms of developing an identity for practitioners that is anything but 'professional'. For better or for worse, many practitioners have framed their identity around this historical process of marginalization; complaints about not being taken seriously, not being valued, not having a voice and sometimes of just being misunderstood abound. While there are, without a doubt, many situations where child and youth care practitioners work collaboratively with other professionals within a context of multi-disciplinary treatment, there are likely far more instances where this is not the case, at least if we ask the child and youth care practitioner. Very often, the articulation of child and youth care practice on the part of practitioners is surprisingly similar to what young people themselves might say about their experience of being cared for; terms such as oppression, under-valuing and peripheral input seem to come up frequently.

A professional identity cannot be built on complaints or feelings of inadequacies. While it is undoubtedly true that there continue to be many issues that hamper the development of child and youth care practice as a full and equal participant along other disciplines in the work with children and youth, it is no longer true that these cannot be addressed unless other systems or other professions initiate change. In fact, at some point in our history as a profession, the balance shifted away from an emphasis on the responsibility of others to open the doors for us to participate toward an emphasis on our responsibility to develop the skills, attitude and capacity to hold our own amongst myriad professions that contribute to a collective effort to make a difference. Our professional identity, therefore, must be built on a foundation that reflects the core principles of child and youth care practice and this identity must be entirely independent of the political context and multi-disciplinary processes and systems in which it exists.

In the chapters throughout this book, I have proposed that our professional identity is based on a number of concepts that remain at the core of what we do regardless of the specific context of our work. Three such core concepts can be captured by the terms caring, engagement and relationship. Regardless of whether we practice in a residential setting or in a school, in the community or in the home of a family or a foster family, our professional endeavor is one that seeks to promote caring as both the experience on the part of the client of being cared for and about as well as the professional activity of giving care and creating caring life spaces. Similarly, the concept of engagement is a necessary and indispensible part of what we do. Every aspect of our work is driven by our engagement of the client and the client's experience of being engaged. The concept of relationship, as the third cornerstone of our practice, ensures that whatever we do and in whatever context we do it, we understand that our practice is based on a mutuality in which we as practitioners are collaborators with our clients and potentially with other professionals in seeking change, growth and meaningful experiences.

It is not particularly difficult to recognize the presence of these concepts in our day to day practice with children, youth and families. As concepts of service provision, caring, engagement and relationship are clearly ever-present and represent what distinguishes our profession from many other helping professions. As I have argued in the foregoing chapters, however, our professional identity should not be limited to situations of direct service. In fact, child and youth care practice represents a specific approach to being with others, whether this is in the context of service provision, program development, policy analysis or management. The skills and professional approaches embedded in child and youth care practice are well suited for a wide range of activities and endeavors, and practitioners must begin to recognize their own competence with respect to leadership positions and taking charge of the process of further developing the field for the better.

As discussed in the chapter on child and youth care approaches to management, virtually the entire spectrum of services for children and youth in which child and youth care practitioners are active have been designed by other professionals following other principles. In Canada, well over one thousand residential programs, hundreds of schools, hospitals and community agencies as well as increasingly early intervention programs, programs and services for homeless or street-involved youth and family preservation programs utilize child and youth care practitioners as a work force to implement pre-determined and pre-packaged approaches to service that very often not only fail to incorporate our principles, but fundamentally contradict these. Issues of power and control, exclusivity and cultural incompetence, one-size fits all philosophies and excessive punitive measures are all prevalent in our workplaces precisely because we have so far failed to take charge of these service settings or contribute meaningfully to all aspects of how they operate. Yet we have plenty to offer. In order to create opportunities for the integration of child and youth care principles into real and existing service settings as well as into policy measures and legislative initiatives, we must use our professional identity with much greater confidence than what we have thus far been able to put forward.

If we can shake off the historical mantel of marginalization and under-valuing of our work, we can use our principles and concepts as well as our approaches to being with children, youth and families in their life spaces as a way of opening the door for programs and services that are inclusive, democratic and meaningful based on the experiences of those we work for and with (the children, youth and families) rather than based exclusively on outcomes generated by a process of number crunching from which we are far removed. In order to do this, of course, we must present ourselves as a credible discipline that has a rightful place in the professions that have long captured the headlines in the children's services sectors.

PROFESSIONAL CONDUCT

In the introduction to this book, I promised to use an eclectic writing style that moved effortlessly from theory to practice and from practice to theory, and I furthermore promised to cover a range of issues from the extremely complex to the seemingly banal. As part of this conclusion to the book, I feel compelled to linger on the seemingly banal for a moment. Professional conduct appears as a self-explanatory variable, one that is simply expected from practitioners seeking greater recognition and value in an already established and highly diversified field of helping professions. I would argue, however, that it is in the area of professional conduct that we, as a collection of practitioners, have met our greatest challenge. Our story of professional conduct begins where our field found its beginnings: in the mayhem of residential group care.

As much as our field has evolved to include positions and activities in myriad contexts and service settings, the vast majority or practitioners in North America in particular continue to be employed in residential group care settings, including residential treatment centres often operated by children's mental health agencies, private residential programs, protection-based programs operated by the child welfare sector, custodial programs operated by the youth justice sector, and education programs operated by either public or private residential schools, boarding schools or other kinds of live-in learning centres. Residential group care is alive and well (or not so well) in the UK and Ireland as well, and in much of Continental Europe, especially in countries such as Germany, Denmark, Belgium and the Netherlands, this mode of intervening with children and youth remains the dominant mode. In Australia and New Zeeland, in spite of much criticism of residential group care and a resurgent focus on family-based care, group homes nevertheless survive, and in Israel and South Africa, children's homes and other kinds of residential group care remain the norm.

The face of our profession, therefore, whether we like it or not, continues to be that of the residential worker, even as we acknowledge the increasing numbers of practitioners who are active in non-residential settings. It is in residential settings more so than anywhere else that child and youth care practitioners have to raise their levels of professional conduct. In spite of the daily challenges associated with the job, and in spite of the imperfect conditions prevalent in most group care settings, practitioners have to move beyond their complacency toward unfortunate incidents, difficult relationships and sometimes unacceptable actions and embrace the idea that their work is based within a theoretical and conceptual framework that calls for much greater thoughtfulness, critical self-evaluation and sophistication in case management and life space intervention techniques. We cannot move forward as a profession so long as we continue to struggle with understanding our presence in the lives of children and youth within the residential setting. The idea that our actions are driven primarily by our own experiences growing up, and perhaps by a rudimentary assessment of what best generates control within the setting and obedience on the part of clients is no longer adequate (it never was, of course). Our professional conduct must be characterized by an on-going curiosity about what we do and why we do this; an unwavering commitment to explore alternative ways of being present and a preparedness to undergo significant and substantive reflective processes and evaluations.

As we raise our level of professional conduct, we also can no longer pretend to not notice those who clearly are not qualified to be amongst us. Every residential practitioner can cite multiple colleagues who are 'burnt out', 'not committed', 'power tripping' or something of that nature. Yet we continue to accept these inadequacies, not realizing that the actions of a few amongst us discredit the work of the many others who in fact are committed to a level of professional conduct worthy of this profession.

The self-regulation of practitioners within residential care settings is especially important because most non-residential practitioners entered the field via the residential sector. It is there where most practitioners adopt their habits within the field. In the absence of a serious commitment to those processes and activities that we know matter most, including attention to the self, commitment to supervision, and an uncompromising endorsement of the concepts of caring, engagement and relationship in everything we do, these practitioners are not very likely to raise their professional conduct once they leave the team context of residential care settings. In fact, in most non-residential contexts in which child and youth care practitioners are employed, the levels of supervision and guidance are significantly reduced, and practitioners therefore will have to rely on their already established habits within their approach to professional conduct even more so than in residential settings.

The rules of professional conduct for child and youth care practitioners are not profoundly different than they are for any other kind of professional; in fact, they ought to be very familiar to the practitioner since much of what constitutes a high level of professional conduct for the practitioner reflects the very expectations we have of the children and youth we work with. It seems reasonable, therefore, to suggest that professional conduct in our field requires the highest possible levels of commitment to problem-solving, reliability and follow through, abstaining from gossip and unconstructive approaches to managing conflict and disagreements as well as contributing to the team (whether it is one of child and youth care practitioners or a multi-disciplinary one) wherever possible and to one's fullest capacity. Professional conduct is closely related to professional competence, and this is the third issue that needs to be addressed.

PROFESSIONAL COMPETENCE

Professional competence in our field has at least two dimensions: one relates to what we actually do, and the other relates to our ability to articulate what we do and why we do it. Child and youth care practice will move forward as a profession when we can claim to be very good in both of these dimensions.

It is no secret to anyone that many practitioners appear to not be very good at this work. Colleagues, children and youth and even supervisors express dismay at their performance. We find non-performers in every profession, and it is in and of itself not particularly worrisome that we also find them in our profession, so long as we can find ways of either raising their performance or gently encouraging a career change. It is much more worrisome that the criteria used to evaluate performance are extremely varied in our field, and can range from the practitioner's ability to exert control over groups of young people to his capacity to engage with one or several youth in relational and meaningful ways. Some of this issue relates to the dominance of other professional training in our supervisory and management ranks. So long as we do not enter those ranks in greater numbers, we will not be able to assert greater focus on our principles and concepts in the evaluation of our performance. Indeed, the under-representation of child and youth care practitioners in positions of leadership in the field is arguably the greatest barrier for the future development of the profession itself. While we can take some comfort in the fact that many leaders in agencies serving children and youth have found their way to our profession, inspired perhaps by our unique focus on relational practice and a commitment to being present in the life spaces of children, youth and their families, this in and of itself is hardly sufficient to carry the profession forward. Ultimately what is needed is a much more systematic approach to thinking about career development in which leadership is one of several possible scenarios.

Issues related to professional competence, however, cannot simply be excused by focusing on external factors. In fact, our tendency to make excuses for professional incompetence is what frequently holds us back as a profession. Seeking professional competence in ourselves and in our child and youth care colleagues must become a priority, with the focus squarely on our own conduct, our own actions and our own decision-making. On the one hand, we can take pride in the fact that our field today produces a great deal of knowledge that can be translated into practice with relative ease. Researchers and conceptual writers in our field now abound, and their work and contributions can help lift us from the periphery of the human services to much more integrated and central positions. For this to happen, however, we will have to take responsibility for actually availing ourselves of this work. In far too many cases, child and youth care practitioners have failed to continue their education and learning once on the job. Blissfully unaware of new thinking and new evidence, they continue to practice in the field using concepts and approaches that were developed decades ago. The focus on behavior, while much criticized at the declaratory level, remains the basis of much of child and youth care practice, especially in residential settings.

While professional competence is certainly of great importance with respect to what we actually do while in the presence of children, youth and families, it is equally important in the context of how we articulate what we do to others. Herein lies another core weakness in our profession. Practitioners often are supremely competent on the job, but they are unable to articulate this to other professionals already predisposed to thinking about our work as banal, clinically unsophisticated or essentially unskilled. In residential care settings, other professionals can at least witness first hand the challenges that present themselves day in and day out, and therefore maintain some level of respect for child and youth care practitioners simply based on their willingness to remain exposed to this apparent chaos. As the profession continues to move outside of residential care, however, the need to be able to articulate clearly what it is we do, why we do it and what the meaning of our work is increases significantly. Child and youth care practitioners have been challenged by professionals in other environments, such as schools for example, where teachers often view their contributions as support functions rather than central components of the learning experience of children and youth. This will not change unless we raise our capacity to articulate what we do more clearly and with greater force and confidence.

CHILD AND YOUTH CARE PRACTICE AND DEMOCRACY

Lest some of the issues cited in this book might leave the impression that our profession is lacking in far too many respects, let me clearly state that child and youth care practice is, although seemingly simple, really very difficult work (Maier, 1985; Phelan, 2008). In many cases we have access to children and youth for only very short periods of time, and only after they have already experienced significant trauma and hardship. Contributing to their developmental growth and preparing them for adulthood is no easy task. The goal of this book was not to point to our inadequacies but rather to highlight the importance of continuing to work hard to improve and enhance what we do every day.

Perhaps the single most important task in moving forward and in ensuring that the inadequacies that do exist are addressed and never complacently accepted as the norm, is that we must re-commit ourselves to a process of being with children, youth and families that is characterized in a fundamental way by the core features of democracy. In this complex project of child and youth care practice, our most important and reliable partners are the children, youth and families themselves. It is not simply a matter of giving them a voice. Our challenge is to re-invent our practice each and every time we encounter a person in need by joining with that person in real and substantive ways. Voice is too easily translated into a token process of input that can be documented. Child and youth are practice is about engaging with people in such a way that their identity, however defined by them, can blossom. It is ultimately about upholding the right of a young person to become someone they can admire and feel good about. It is not the goal of child and youth care practice to impose onto young persons a set of skills and attributes that equip them merely to become what we envision for them. Only under conditions of democracy, whereby worker and child become a relationally connected force for change, can our project lay claim to its lofty ambitions.

REFERENCES

Bettelheim, B. (1974). *A home for the heart.* New York: Alfred A. Knopf.

Brendtro, L., Brokenleg, M., & VanB, S. (1990). *Reclaiming youth at risk: Our hope for the future.* Bloomington, IN: National Education Service.

Brendtro, L., Ness, A., & Mitchell, M. (2005). *No disposable kids.* Bloomington, IN: National Education Service.

Maier, H.W. (1985). Primary care in secondary settings: inherent strains, in Fulcher, L. C. and Ainsworth, F. (1985) *Group Care Practice with Children.* London: Tavistock.

Phelan, J. (2008). Living with complexity and simplicity. *CYC OnLine,* Issue 109. Retrieved on March 23, 2010 from http://www.cyc-net.org/cyc-online/cycol-0308-phelan.html

Redl, F., & Wineman, D. (1952). *Controls from within: Techniques for the treatment of the aggressive child.* Glencoe, IL: Free Press.

Index